The Energy Connection

Answers to life's important questions

Betty F. Balcombe

PIATKUS

To all who have helped make
this book possible by
continuously
asking for more.

© 1993 B F Balcombe

First published in 1993 by
Judy Piatkus (Publishers) Ltd of
5 Windmill Street, London W1P 1HF

**The moral right of the author
has been asserted**

*A catalogue record for this book is
available from the British Library*

ISBN 0 – 7499 – 1217 – 0

Edited by Martin Noble
Designed by Sue Ryall
Illustrations by Zena Flax

Set in 12/14pt Compugraphic Baskerville by
Action Typesetting, Gloucester
Printed and bound in Great Britain by
Mackays of Chatham PLC

Contents

Part II: ENERGY

Part III: HEALING AND AURA ENERGY

Part IV: CEREMONIES

Part V: QUESTIONS AND ANSWERS   183

Introduction

I have been aware of my 'oddness' and sense of 'difference' since I was a child but gradually learned to understand and integrate with people although I often found them very strange and muddled! They were, in turn, sometimes afraid of me and at other times tried to accept me and my 'strangeness'! I 'saw' colours and energies, 'knew' about people and their problems, and felt healing energy transferring from me to them when they had a need.

Eventually, through searching my inner self and questioning avidly everyone I met who had a theory about psychics and spiritual awareness, I found who and what I am. I am what is known as a psychic. This means that I am able to give healing energy to people who have an energy imbalance and are unwell, in order that they can help themselves. It also means I am able to tune into the aura field which surrounds us all as individuals, and translate what is received. This I do to help those in trouble and confusion in order that they can understand and choose their path in life.

By the time I reached my teens I was giving 'readings' to anyone who asked. I found, by gazing at them or any object near by, I was able to tell them about themselves and what their actions were leading them to. I used and developed this ability and combined healing energy sessions and readings to find the cause of illness or imbalance.

Eventually I was asked if I would teach what I had learned and what I practised. And so my classes for psychic and spiritual development began.

As the years have passed by I have practised my philosophy of life. I believe all reasoning beings have the right to knowledge, that no one has the perfect way of life for all and that we need to question and search our inner senses, physical knowledge, spiritual connection and soul wisdom, to find our own path in life. We do this by debate, exchange of ideas, theories and insights. Communication is needed to remove fear, and by removing fear we free our thoughts.

In 1988 I wrote my first book *As I See It* .... I wrote it at the request of those who had been to my classes for psychic and spiritual development and those who had been to see me over the years either for help or because they were interested in learning more about my ideas and philosophy.

Via these people and the 'grapevine', *As I See It* ... has been purchased by people all over the world. It was originally intended as a private publication for those who knew of me but it has now been read by many who have not met me personally but seek clarity about a subject which is full of antiquated ideas, fear and muddle.

Since *As I See It* ... was published I have received so many requests for more that I decided to write my second book, *The Energy Connection*.

The Energy Connection is a part of the quest for clarity and the removal of prejudice and fear which still surrounds psychic and spiritual matters. As well as incorporating the answers to questions and requests from friends, students and readers for further information, this book also includes material from spontaneous talks I have given which were recorded at the time and then transcribed.

My aim is to take you, the reader, on a gentle journey through a variety of subjects. The common thread is energy as the life force. I have divided the book into four main sections because it flows more naturally this way and each section forms a stepping stone to the next which gives resting spaces to pause and think.

I have covered a great deal of subject matter in this book, ranging from 'The Three Levels of Life' to 'Ending a Physical Life', and from 'Energy Communication' to the 'Energy Underlying Numbers'. I have written about healing energy and combining energy to celebrate, and I end by answering questions I am often asked and thought would be of interest to others.

Gathering together the thoughts, notes, questions and ideas for this book has been very joyful to me. I give them now to you, and hope that you enjoy your walk through them as much as I have enjoyed writing them.

Betty F. Balcombe

Preface

Our spirit is our life-force for the duration of a life on earth. Our soul is our overself, our true self, and is always in contact with our spirit.

We are three-stage beings while on Earth; a soul, a spirit and a physical body. Together they are our whole being and to honour our total self we need to look after each of them, giving each level respect, dignity and care in order to be able to extend to others and show, by example, that life can be beautiful and manageable, if we practise care and responsibility. When we do not honour ourselves, our energy fades and we become unseeable.

Life may not always be wonderful or kind; it can even be cruel and feel unjust, but we are part of all that happens to us and others. When we find our own inner stillness and believe in our right to live in peace and dignity, we will overcome all obstacles and help others to do the same.

Practice does not make perfect – practice makes possible.

Part I

Communication

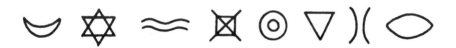

1
Communication

Sharing experiences, speaking and listening are essential in order that we can expand and become balanced. How we approach this harvest is important.

With knowledge and understanding comes the strength and ability to select the best road to follow at any one time. Our needs change as we progress through life. We add to our store of knowledge, absorbing and expanding to incorporate all that a new line of energy offers us; or we stay afraid, unmoving, clinging on to other people and the needs of yesterday.

A course of lessons should stimulate, allow questions, give understandable answers, be logical, beneficial and be something that we can give and receive from. All things learned should be shared. Any course specifically for the spiritual self should incorporate the physical self and vice versa. They cannot be separated. They need each other to exist. If we are in harmony, we communicate harmony to others. If we are out of harmony, we can smile, give advice and appear to listen, but the energy we emit will be lacking in quality and substance and this will be sensed by others, causing confusion.

We sense much more when we are calm and alert when speaking or listening. When we constantly talk, we give little and hear less. Being calm and alert enables us to pause to formulate questions and answer them. The energy we emit will come from our own source and need for knowledge. Persistently insisting we are correct does not make a truth. People who are unsure of their subject, or are full of what they believe to be a truth, are afraid of questions in case their belief has flaws, which they are unwilling to acknowledge. Those who have achieved inner harmony and peace are open to debate because they know there is always something to add to knowledge and are willing to hear other views. They are interested in questions and answers and can afford to listen. If we are quietly active within our own space and observe, we are able to sense the energy behind the words and can then make a contribution which has meaning.

We all have knowledge and experiences to share. We absorb all the time as we, sometimes unknowingly, watch others through our life. Some people rarely speak because they are afraid to express an opinion in case they seem ignorant or others might laugh at them. They have knowledge and experiences to share but keep them hidden. If we hold on to everything we learn or experience, our ability to assess what we have collected is limited.

Humans in their natural state have a very strong survival instinct. A baby and the young child are very survival-conscious. If we observe a young child we will notice that they lift their head, almost sniffing the air, before they go into a room. When they go to a new place or meet new people, they stand at the doorway or near a person they trust. They are not shy, as some think; they are listening and sensing the sound of the place and people to see if it is safe to enter. If they are not allowed that moment to acclimatise and are forced too quickly to join in, their behaviour can become withdrawn or over-active. If they can communicate with the energy around them, pause and sense the atmosphere, they will usually enter quietly in a short while. They know whom they can trust by sense.

A great many of our thoughts are filled with fear because we lack communication with others. Ideas and theories from various sources can be stimulating, but if they are communicated as truths only because they have lasted for years they can be misleading. Many are rewritten and added to over the years, eventually becoming what others believed was meant, not what was actually said.

Theories and opinions can change with added knowledge, and questioning shows their strengths and weaknesses. An idea or theory does not become a truth because it has lasted by being repeated down the ages, or because the speaker is well known or erudite.

Theories change as time passes and the common and individual consciousness of humankind expands. Expansion and understanding are impossible if we do not allow old beliefs to be examined in the light of today's knowledge. Information and understanding change constantly and what was acceptable or not acceptable in the past can be re-assessed.

The speaker makes available an idea; the listener questions, accepts or rejects. All need to question and answer each other. That is expansion.

Due to lack of open minds, debate laced with prejudice and pre-formed opinions, certain words and subjects have caused fear and terror in many people, and still do.

How we use words is very important. Words are energy and create thought-forms. They can trigger imagination, fear, excitement, depression, joy or well-being.

FEAR

It is very easy to get an unbalanced view of the world. Newspapers and the media constantly report the terror, cruelty and the catastrophies of life. A person whose job it is to help the sick, frightened and those unable to cope, constantly hears the fears and worries of everyday life. It can seem to us all at times that society is full of weak, frightened, ill-treated people and misery of one kind or another. There is more cruelty and fear, because we have multiplied and also because we are living in closer proximity to each other. We are all afraid of being invaded and attacked by people and situations, and the more we own and live close to each other the more we are afraid of loss. Fear is contagious and spreads at an alarming rate. There is also the opposite which means the more of us there are, the more we can do positively. There is also more care and understanding which can be communicated if we allow ourselves to use it.

The fear energy we emit feeds the type of people and situations we are afraid of, who thrive on that fear energy, absorbing it to become stronger. This type of energy exchange is not only person-to-person but reaches out into society. The potential victims feed the potential aggressors. Fear feeds what we are afraid of. Communication energy, however, can also be uplifting and life-giving. Energy does not choose its nature and quality, humans affect it and use it. The world is not to blame for our troubles, it is people. Listen and spread the good news; there are millions of people who care, actively using their energy to try and improve the quality of life.

CARE

Many of us speak without any care at all as to where our thoughts began, where our words are going, or the effect they have on someone else. For instance, there are the people who are constantly apologising, when what has occurred has nothing to do with them. This removes the right of the person who is truly involved to clear their path. There is also the throw-away phrase 'Take care of yourself', which is tossed at someone with no caring thought at all and they are immediately forgotten. Sending such a request with the energy of care is a warm and comforting gift. When it is given without energy, it becomes dismissive.

PSYCHICS AND PSYCHIC ENERGY

The word 'psychic' causes a great deal of fear in those who do not have knowledge or understanding.

A person who is psychic has an extra energy and the ability to give that extra energy to others so that they can heal themselves. Psychics can also 'see', 'sense' or 'know' certain information about another person. It is a natural ability and the psychic energy can be communicated in many other ways, manifesting through music, art, performing, writing, the caring professions and communication in all its diversity. Many psychics are unaware that they have this extra energy until something unusual occurs to draw it to their attention. Psychics are not special, but they are different. This can cause them imbalance and fear if they do not understand what makes them different. It can also cause fear in others if they sense the difference and cannot find a rational explanation for it.

Psychics are ordinary people with ordinary, everday needs and, like all others, they need to sleep, wash, eat, dress; they have mood-swings, upsets, inflated egos, likes, dislikes; they make mistakes, do wonderful things, are kind, greedy, loving, cruel; are wise, stupid, self-opinionated, have low or high self-esteem. Psychics are no different in these ways to everyone else. Being spiritual does not mean that a person is psychic, any more than being psychic means that a person is spiritual. A psychic can be totally self-absorbed or open and caring. They can use their ability to help others to achieve self-responsibility and strength of mind; they can, through promises, threats and/or fear, attract weak people, frightening them into obedience. Some people follow a psychic because they radiate light and energy, offering knowledge of a better way of life. A psychic can fascinate by their voice, whatever the content of their communication. Some psychics are very spiritual, honest and caring, having reached an awareness of their energy and the responsibility that goes with it.

A great many psychics use their ability to heal and communicate on many levels and are accepted because they are seen to live life in a clear and acceptable way. They do not profess to be what they are not, and show care for quality of life and health, in the mind, body and spirit. They will discuss and answer questions about their work.

No-one has spiritual power over someone else, but we can feed another person energy by believing they have superior power and thereby choosing to submit to their commands. That is our choice. All beings have their own inner power and can choose how they use it. However strong in vitality, energy and the ability to speak well a person is, they cannot have power over someone else unless that other person chooses to believe and agrees to contribute.

Some psychics give messages to other people purported to come from spirits or spiritual beings.

CHANNELLING

The word 'channelling' is very widely used. It usually means information from a source outside the speaker and not part of them. However, the word does not convey the information of where the voice or message is coming from. It is foolish to assume that everything that comes along a channel or is passed through a channel is from a highly evolved soul, or that the information is worth while.

A strangely accented voice speaking through a person called a 'channeller' should be questioned as to why it needs an accent. If the channeller speaks without one, the accent can be an affectation. If the voice is of someone who is physically dead, but was known in life and had an accent, this can be proof of connection. A soul does not have to take language lessons to communicate. It will use a language known in a past life or the one used by the channeller in this lifetime. The 'communicator' should be questioned as to who, what and where they are.

Some seemingly channelled communications arise from the subconscious desire of the speaker to attract attention. Some voices are a cover, used by the psychic who is able to sense and convey genuine information to people, but the information is more potent and acceptable by listeners if it is conveyed in a foreign-sounding accent said to be a guide or a highly evolved soul. This practice enables the medium/psychic to appear detached and not responsible for what is said. This can all be carried out unconsciously or purposefully.

There are people who can communicate via their spirit and soul connection in a beautiful, profound and inspired way in their own voice, knowing exactly what they are saying and taking responsibility for their words. There are others who communicate in this way who are not aware of what is said, but the quality of the communication is clear and, in most cases, questions are welcomed and answered. These communications are outstanding in quality and to the point. They do not threaten, do not stress any religions or beliefs, but attempt to connect the listeners to their own soul and inner wonder, putting responsibility firmly back where it belongs.

Any information purported to be from a spirit or spiritual being should be handled with care by the giver and receiver. True higher soul communication will encourage choice, free will and self-responsibility. Information which is personal is usually obtained from our own spirit, soul or past-life experience. Most people find it hard to acknowledge the wonder of our own souls. They are quite happy to accept communication if it is said to come from a higher energy than themselves, but cannot accept wisdom from their own source. What we seem to be physically, mentally and spiritually in this life is not always an indication of what has been achieved in knowledge and wisdom by our soul. It is natural for our overself, our soul, to communicate with us through our own spirit via our physical senses.

When we are given information which has depth of meaning and beauty, it does not have to be from some other being. We communicate with our three-fold self – the soul, the spirit, the physical – and we would understand and harmonise better with each other and life if we could acknowledge that we all have the potential to be wonderful beings. We have been physically alive on this planet for millions of years and have been evolving as souls for all that time. If we accept the magnitude and marvel of this ongoing wonder, we would stand straighter and live up to our greatness.

'OCCULT' AND 'MAGIC'

Many people are terrified of the words 'occult' and 'magic'. They are full of fear and superstition, but little knowledge. This fear of the unknown is encouraged, and those who love power over others wrap these subjects in mystery for their own purposes.

First of all, the basic meaning of words needs to be understood in order to get a perspective. According to dictionaries:

Occult means: to be hidden, unknown;
Magic means: unaccountable or baffling effects.

Surely this constitutes a challenge to find out more, not behave like the ostrich.

Many things have been called 'occult' and 'magic' in bygone times which are now acceptable and absorbed into our everyday lives. In other societies in countries throughout the world, what is acceptable to us would seem like magic to them: aeroplanes, telephones, television, photographs, electricity can all cause fear in those who do not understand. When they are explained, the ear of the unknown, unaccountable or baffling effects disappears.

We are afraid of the 'magic' from other cultures just as they are afraid of ours: spells, curses, moving inanimate objects, causing weather to change, are all alien to our minds. To other cultures they are normal, understood and acceptable. Until we investigate and gain understanding we will remain frightened of each other and life.

We are all afraid of the unknown at some time, the hidden, secret fears we try to ignore, but with sharing and communication, debate and understanding, we can shed light on taboo subjects. Those people who prey on the fear in others, and make money out of the distress to which they contribute, will then find it very hard to continue.

Whether the lack of understanding is about words, abilities, power, beliefs or mechanical objects, misunderstandings can be removed. When the hidden is seen and understood, the unknown investigated, the unaccountable or baffling discussed, those things which caused deep fear become interesting and usable. All things are energy and can be explained. Because we cannot explain all things now, through our lack of knowledge and communication, does not mean there are no answers.

ADDICTION

Life's energies can go out of balance in all of us at times and addiction is an imbalance in a person's energy field. The word 'addict' is used as a label for many people who are out of control in relation to certain substances or behaviour. We are inclined to see addiction as a weakness in others.

Addiction is a human characteristic. All humans can be, and are, addicted in various ways. In the majority of cases, the need is channelled into another person, work, religion, an idea, object, sport or a hobby. These people do not see themselves as addicts, but removal of their focal point could cause them to have withdrawal symptoms, often losing interest in living and self-care, just as other 'addicts' do.

Some addictions are harmless to the person concerned and others, but some are very dangerous and not only impair the life and well-being of the addict, but also other people.

If a person is addicted to a self-destroying substance, taking them off their chosen desire causes crises on all levels. They need care, understanding, weaning away and to have something else to replace the addiction. Before the weaning commences, the replacement should be introduced, making sure the replacement is constructive, not destructive.

We all have the potential to be addicted to something and should acknowledge that fact, and so understand and care about those whose addictions have become life-consuming and are considered anti-social.

NEGATIVE ENERGY AND POSSESSION

Some people are told that their behaviour is caused by an 'entity' or that they are 'possessed'.

The word 'possession' is used by those who believe there are evil spirits in the atmosphere which take over any unwary persons. There are no spirits, evil or not, lurking ready to pounce. Spirit energy is either connected to its physical body base or with its soul.

The energies which surround us and affect us all are created by our own actions on Earth as physical beings. This human energy can be transmitted and accepted consciously or subconsciously. When we work or live in an unsuitable environment, in fearful conditions, or with depressed or frightened people, we can pick up via our aura the essence of these energies. However we also constantly and naturally repel all that is alien to our own aura while we are well and feel in control. Should our energy become low through constant exposure to unsuitable situations, we attract negative energy from others and hold on to it. We can then add to it our own fear through what we watch, read and the company we keep. This negative essence can gradually build up in our electro-magnetic aura layer which is close to our physical body and this can affect our behaviour and thinking. (See pages 148 – 166 on aura energy.) Possession is not the spirit of another person, but is our tendency to allow alien energy to build up around us and feed it with our own fears and desires.

AURA CLEARING

A psychic would see this alien enegy as a deep, dark blue which can appear black, mainly around the head and shoulders of the person, sometimes slightly to one side. This is because it is causing an imbalance in the aura. Aura clearing, plus psychic attunement with the person to locate the causes of the build-up, are the first steps to be carried out. The person who is affected and behaving in an unacceptable or uncharacteristic way will also have to want to make changes in their life, to remove themself from the causes, as soon as possible, wherever the energy build-up is from – home, work, environment or self-inflicted by watching or taking part in activities which are unacceptable to their spirit. All that affects the physical is recorded in the aura and affects the spirit; all that is recorded by the spirit affects the physical. All energies transmitted from each of us affect all of us.

BLOCKAGES

Some words are used a great deal to explain imbalance and confusion. Not all people translate them the same. When a person is told that they are 'blocked' in one of their centres (see pages 30 – 34 on the energy centres), it triggers the image of a complete stoppage and the feeling of being 'blocked' is intensified or created. This can then cause a minor imbalance to become a major problem.

It is not possible to 'block' a centre in a living creature. The centre can be under-energised or over-energised. It can be intensely or weakly affecting the aura energy but it cannot be 'blocked'.

15

An emotional disaster will not cause energy to stop. It will unbalance the emotional centre and all other centre energies will then be affected, as all centres are represented in all others. A person told that their lack of love is caused by a 'blockage' in their emotional centre could use that as a reason for their loneliness, accepting the label and not doing anything to improve the situation. Loving starts from within, with the acceptance that we can all love and are lovable, whatever shape, colour or size we are. If a person feels unloved, or unloving, they can be helped by counselling and healing energy. The start of loving is healing and until the person is strong enough to heal themselves, a carer can give them the help and energy they need to strengthen and calm the centre.

'UNGROUNDED'

'Ungrounded' is another word we constantly hear which can be translated many ways. When a person feels unreal and is unable to cope within the reality of life, they are often told they are 'ungrounded'. The unreal feeling can also be caused because they are *too much* in touch with reality and their inner self-defence energy has switched them into non-connection. They need to check how deeply involved they are with material things.

Some people feel unreal due to deficiencies and should check their diet. Deficiency can cause light-headedness or disconnection, and hallucinations can occur when people speak of hearing voices telling them what to do. Disconnection can also occur during an emotionally charged situation such as group chanting or meditation. On these occasions, some people extend their consciousness which can seem like an out-of-body experience. They can enjoy this state so much they try to keep it, living in a half-world as in a dream. They lose touch with reality on Earth and do not want, or have forgotten, to see life through their physical eyes.

This state is often confused with out-of-body experiences. When the spirit leaves the body, the person cannot move and thinking is with the spirit. If, therefore, they are conscious of self and able to move physically, but feel above or outside themselves, this is a state of extended or expanded consciousness. They are experiencing through their aura energy via their physical. This causes vagueness, an inability to make choices or decisions and can enable them to observe themselves in a detached way from a point outside their body, even hearing their physical self speaking as though they were a separate person and not responsible for the words being spoken by their physical self.

In certain circumstances a person can be under-active in one of their centres. This creates a feeling of detachment and/or emptiness.

THE USE AND MISUSE OF LANGUAGE

Words are often used without understanding and care, without energy input, without thought. Many people argue a point when they actually agree with each other, but their use of words gives an impression they are on opposite sides.

If a statement has been made, there is no need to repeat it afterwards another way. The dreaded phrase 'in other words' brings a chill to many of us and clarity can turn into confusion with the second and third explanation.

If we attend a meeting, lecture or workshop, or have a private session with someone, we should make sure we understand what they mean. Asking another person afterwards what they thought was meant results in an opinion, not an answer. Ask the speaker questions and listen to the answers. If necessary, ask more questions until understanding is achieved. No-one is too elevated to be questioned. We know what we know by the questions we can answer.

A profound statement reaches below surface thought and the obvious. This does not mean it should be impossible to understand. Its profundity, its depth, should reach out in clarity. If understanding is impossible and the sense buried, it does not mean it is a profound statement. A person who speaks in riddles or communicates in a way we cannot understand is not always 'deep'.

In-depth thinking and communication removes covers and subterfuges as it reaches the spirit and resounds from the soul.

If a speaker is difficult to understand, we should not assume we are less intelligent or lacking in spiritual evolvement. Seek clarity and thereby expand the understanding of both the listeners and the speaker.

Stating that certain things are right or wrong does not make them so, or mean that we have understanding of others and what they are involved in or believe. A person can say and feel things are right or wrong, but may not question their reasons for feeling this way. If we use, instead, the words 'acceptable' and 'unacceptable', we can make all things personal, and action and understanding are possible.

If words and actions are repeated often enough they can be absorbed and become patterns accepted by us and our society, usually with very little questioning or understanding. If another country or society has a different way of living, we are quick to condemn, be frightened, and even attack, because the difference in the energy pattern stands out and does not fit our own. We say they are wrong and we are right. This leads to lack of understanding, cruelty, oppression and conflict. By discussing our differences we will all benefit from ideas, knowledge exchanged, and can find understanding if not acceptance. No person or country has discovered the best way to live for all, only their own way created for themselves from their history and beliefs. It does not mean one system is 'right' and another 'wrong'. Many humans do not acknowledge others from different backgrounds and cultures as equal to themselves, and each culture fears the other, feeling they are right and the others are wrong.

If we could each acknowledge we are not yet perfect, and do not know what is best for everyone else, we could learn from each other and be brave enough to admit we do not know all the answers to all the questions of living on this planet. We would then be in a better position to listen and exchange, which would put us one step forward toward becoming Human Beings.

We should not believe in something because somebody says it is true, or believe in traditions because they have been handed down through the ages. We should not believe written things just because they were written long ago. Nor should we accept as true the words of supposedly spiritual beings, however their message is received. We should not follow instructions or orders when our reasoning and senses doubt their truth.

We need to listen, think, and above all sense what is acceptable to us from our own experiences. Humankind is unique on this planet. There is no other life form on Earth that has the ability to reason as we do.

Machinery only works as long as energy is fed into it. Humans are required to set this chain of events in motion and maintain it. Our energy makes things happen. We are responsible for our energy. If we do not acknowledge our vast energy flow and use it wisely, we will continue to destroy creatures, cultures, each other, and the Earth.

Communication on all levels, through music, art, dance, literature, film, is vital energy and we choose the quality of that energy in our lives by what we choose to absorb and accept.

Words are our everyday communication energy. Too many or too few cause fear and misunderstanding. The listener is as important as the speaker and regulates by questions what quality of word energy is received and shared by us all. The quality of life improves with the quality of communication.

In the air around us are waves of sound energy being transmitted from many sources. Sound energy which comes from a caring source creates harmony. Sound energy from disharmony and confusion transmits chaos and fear and we are all affected. At times there is complete sound chaos around us as the air waves become full of TV, radio and people noises, causing confusion, stress and anger in all of us. In the early hours of the morning a great peace can be experienced by those awake for all the electricity and noise around us has lessened considerably and the atmosphere seems clear and magical. As the sun rises we feel inspired, and in communication with life within us and around us.

2
The Three Levels of Life: Soul, Spirit, Physical

Our souls choose to be part of a physical experience on Earth and, during that physical experience, contribute via the spirit to the combined consciousness of humankind. The physical body is inherited and incorporates memories and patterns of all people who have gone into its making down the ages.

Our spirit shines through our aura and is part of, and always in connection with, our soul. The soul does not come to Earth. It is based in the spiral of energy which is around the planet. The soul evolves via lives on Earth and a life as a soul. Each soul is individual, but not individualistic, and is a complete record of our existence since life began on the planet aeons ago. It is made up of all our past-life experiences. When we need help and experience we receive this via our spirit, from our soul. The spirit is a reflection and is part of the soul, and resides in the physical body during its stay on Earth.

As three-stage beings, a soul, a spirit and a physical, it is how we blend and co-ordinate these three that is important. We do not inherit our soul from others. It is our true self, our completeness. Memories of our many lives and experiences on Earth add to our soul energy which strives to be responsible for itself, using all experiences gained to progress. All of space is full of life, the life of souls. Our soul life energy is around our own planet Earth.

Our soul life is our reality; our spirit is a part of, and an energy reflection from, our soul, which chooses to have a physical experience on Earth and therefore needs a physical body to live in. The physical body energy field enables the spirit to interrelate, experience and be in touch with all other things physical. However, our physical body is inherited from our parents. They inherited their bodies from four others and the chain reaches far back in time. We also inherit the genetic coding of all ancestors. This physical inheritance can have faults and imperfections in its brain, body and mental processes.

We have a clear line of experience and memory from our soul in our physical life, which is not inherited from others. The soul is the total of all its own experiences.

PHYSICAL

While on Earth we are part of our soul and able to contact it at all times via our spirit energy. We gradually forget our soul past at birth. As we become adult we become puzzled and lost, wondering what life is all about, constantly losing touch with our greater self. We live as a fragment of our whole self instead of acknowledging ourselves as part of its greatness. When we acknowledge we are part of our soul we cannot be small-minded, we cannot behave inhumanely. Because we keep living at the level of our physical smallness and fears, we harm ourselves and each other. If we all reached inwards to our spirit and up to our soul energy, we would reach our greater potential and the common consciousness of the planet would shift, enabling all of us to benefit.

Humans are not yet Human Beings. While we behave in an uncaring way to each other and the planet, we are proving that we have not reached Being status and cannot call ourselves Human Beings. Because we believe we have reached our zenith, we do not feel we have to try hard. By admitting we have much to learn, we can expand and explore, remove props and become true to ourselves. Rules and laws only work if we all agree to abide by them. This applies to personal structures as well. We need to check periodically to see if they reflect our present needs. Each of us is important and different and a part of a greater pattern. We are not repeats or copies of others, but are a new mixture. With each new life we are in a different physical body and the world and its societies are also different. Life on Earth does not stand still while our spirit is away from its soul; all people and life on Earth continually change. We have to relearn how to live each time we come here; with different bodies, families, friends and society. We make decisions and plans regarding our life and environment, while we are on Earth. Life is not mapped out in advance. We have free will. We are not bound by past lives they are experiences gained from lives completed, however incomplete or unacceptable they seem to us now.

We learn from each other while on Earth, accumulating ideas and patterns which belong to others. We learn about war; some people are born with the genetic or historical memory of soldiering and battle. This does not make war inevitable. Thinking creates an energy and a conscious dream creates the energy of reality, for construction or destruction. We can, therefore, create the thought-form that can cause wars. When two countries have a dispute, there are people who immediately think and say that war is inevitable. They are creating an energy which links into the common memory which is all around us of past wars, and gradually others tune into the war memory and add to it. The war which need not be becomes the war which is inevitable. The energy created by the dispute is fed by the energy of the fear of war and war becomes a reality.

We can refuse to join in the war thought-form and talk of peace and negotiate, so that we can begin to neutralise the energy of the thought-form of war and the war can be averted. Having thoughts of a war-less planet and working towards that dream will make it a reality.

Many people meditate and think of peace and understanding, which encourages harmony in the world. Positive thought energy coupled with interaction does achieve results. Many disputes and dangerous situations have been averted through debate. We can see the results around us, from friends, families, neighbours and, in a greater way, between countries. We are all conscious of the power of thought and speech.

If we acknowledge we have inherited patterns and can change, mould and use the best, we get a taste of what we can achieve, firstly as individuals and then as communities.

Looking after our basic needs is not selfish. Nor is it selfish to attend to our inner self so long as we help others to do the same. Everyone is special and different and all are individual. Each of us is no better or worse than anybody else. At times we feel really wonderful and at other times worthless, but we are still very special beings. Each of us has a role to play in achieving harmony with all things. Some people believe we are like grains of sand on the beach and are individually worthless; but if every grain of sand was individually removed from the beach, there would eventually not be a beach. Every grain of sand is important and contributes to the whole, just as humans do to life on Earth.

Life has patterns. Patterns keep each person in harmony and these patterns, when acknowledged and used, show us the simplicity of life. We are afraid of the nudity of simplicity; afraid to look life in the eye, seeing its wonder. We tune into fear, wrap simplicity up and hide it away, and the fear causes havoc and imbalance with no check. If we could be a little braver, then we would not find life so difficult because we would look at who and what we are, asking ourselves questions on where the difficulties come from. If life seems to be in chaos and a solution is hard to find because everything seems to have gone wrong, seek the source of confusion. Many of us think we have problems when we are really taking the troubles of others on to our shoulders instead of helping them solve their own.

Loss of self-worth can occur when we try to live up to the expectations of others. We have a choice, to live to patterns someone else has laid down for us or to construct and use our own patterns.

If we ask someone what they think of us, we are giving them permission to give us an opinion. We should not then feel hurt and angry if we do not like what they say. Many of us inadvertently put ourselves in a self-deprecating pattern.

When our way of life is such that it does not interfere with the harmony of others, we are in harmony ourselves. If we allow unacceptable behaviour to fill the space of other people, disturbing, hurting and destroying them, we are doing the same to ourselves. The human body energy comes from various sources; our soul energy connecting via our spirit; from movement of the body; our food intake; the air we breathe and the company we keep. All energy received is usable and needs to be replenished. Energy cannot be stored. A person who rests continuously loses the means to move. A person who moves rhythmically will find they become tireless. A car battery is similar. If the car is used regularly, the battery will recharge itself. If the car is unused, the battery will become flat and lifeless. It is better for a person to be encouraged to move, even a finger, than to be immobile. This applies to the spirit as well as the physical.

SPIRIT

When a person feels the need to contact and understand their spirituality, they also need to be aware of their physical life and their contribution to all life on the planet. For the spirit to evolve on Earth, it has to incorporate the physical existence. To refine our spirit we have to work on our physical involvement in life first. They go hand in hand. Shutting out reality and isolating ourselves from what is disharmonious around us in the world is not a growth process for the spirit or the physical. A truly integrated being lives the physical life, using spiritual values, in connection with their soul. Refinement of the spirit energy involves all we do on all levels of life.

When our spirit returns to its soul at our physical dying time, it is returning to its true self to become absorbed in the whole. The physical life just ended has to be cleared and completed. The soul cannot absorb its spirit energy and all it has been involved in on Earth until understanding and harmony have been achieved.

The spirit, as part of a physical existence, has experienced and been involved in many situations. If the physical life was short and ended as a child, the absorbtion is immediate. Some souls choose another physical existence quite quickly in these circumstances.

The soul senses the physical life its spirit has just completed in its entirety. It contacts the essence of the life, sifting, recording and finally absorbing all that has been learned and experienced. All activity during the Earth life is sensed. The spirit has to face and clear everything it has been involved in, during its physical existence. Although the brain and mind may have been in control and its use of the body caused the pain to others, the spirit has still recorded the events and must clear them. The spirit has no capacity to pass blame on to circumstances or others. The soul receives knowledge of the life just left as it is lived, and it is now in a position to see and sense it as a whole, from all angles. The spirit was involved in all actions, whether willingly or not, and will be responsible for clearing all that happened which is unacceptable.

SOUL

The soul is not a judge and jury, it is an overseer, responsible for the actions of all aspects of itself. Clarification and understanding have to be achieved in relation to the life just completed. The spirit needs the opportunity to meet those affected in order to become part of its soul.

The spirit and soul need to come to terms with all that happened and to gain understanding from others still on Earth or already with their soul. With understanding, the spirit can forgive itself or come to terms with its last life involvement. The soul, via its spirit, works to get the understanding needed so all concerned can absorb and progress. When harmony is achieved, the spirit is absorbed into its soul. The memory of the life just ended is now part of the soul, the real self.

The memories of all past lives add to the character and knowledge of the soul. Each soul has an individual personality and identity. The soul's gentleness is a part of its spirit energy which, at times, finds difficulty in shining through during a physical life. The spirit energy is a part and a reflection of its soul. Harmony and understanding between the two essences on the return of the spirit is essential, as the spirit has been involved in physical experiences which can change its vibration and therefore its energy.

When the spirit returns to its soul, it is actually going home. If the pre-chosen time to return has arrived, the physical is no longer needed. When the spirit reaches its soul it not only recalls a life involvement through the physical brain and body, but as the soul recorded them. Although the spirit is responsible for clearing all that happened, it also takes into account the environment, education, background and influences of others while it was on Earth.

At times, when the brain via the mind does not listen to the spirit, it cannot then guide and nourish. Brain energy is very strong and can take almost complete control of a life. When this happens, the person is like a robot, responding without thought, acting without compassion. Spirits remembering the last life recall good, funny, sad and beautiful memories, as well as those it would rather had not occurred. It sees the rough and tumble of being human as part of a whole pattern.

One way a spirit can contact with a person still on Earth once it is with its soul is through dreams. The living person dreams of meeting someone they hated or feared, who has physically died, and is able, via this process, to release pain and anger. The visiting spirit puts its case, seeking understanding for what occurred while as a physical being on Earth. The soul and spirit see clearly without a brain's interference, and the spirit attempts to get the dreamer who was harmed to understand too. Once that understanding is reached, they can forgive themselves. If that understanding is not given, the soul and spirit will wait and try again when the physical person is older. When understanding cannot be reached via this process, depending on the disruption caused, the soul will accept its spirit and deal with the matter when the living person dies and its spirit is free to clarify for itself.

The soul moves through the energy of evolution to suit its vibration and refinement. It is a gradual process of change. As souls we meet others of compatible vibration. We evolve, but need to keep in touch with the whole essence of life. When living on the Earth as a physical being with spirit energy, we meet spirits from many levels of soul evolution. This is why the people we meet are so different; their spirits come from different souls and their bodies have inherited a vast amount from centuries of forebears.

THE THREE LEVELS

The planet Earth is a wonderful place. It also has a soul and spirit. It holds every energy, every idea, every thought from every source, since time began. We are affected by those memories, the acceptable and unacceptable. If we look at the planet as a great garden, we can see that some of it seems wild and barren and other parts seem light and fragrant. The people are the plants and can choke and destroy or be beautifying and uplifting, adding beauty to the garden. We learn to adjust to the differences of life, not to judge but to sense the inner energy and spirit of the planet and people.

We can help each other and help our souls and, by being aware of life, adding to it, we learn about all levels of soul and each other. It is very important how we behave on Earth as we affect the whole universe.

While on Earth the essence of our spirit rests in our solar centre when in harmony. It is directly connected to the spirit energy centre called Kundalini, and the golden bowl centre called soul connection. It is, therefore, always in contact with its soul. The Kundalini centre is located at the base of the nerve centre, which is also called the tree of life and runs parallel with the spine, linking all energy centres and physical centres to each other. The soul connection centre is based in the top of the skull.

All energies, via soul, spirit and physical, are linked and need each other to function well on all levels. Many people do not realise the wonderful, simple beauty of this natural process. It does not need years of work to achieve. It is not the prerogative of the few. It does not need initiation ceremonies or elitist company. It is the right and natural state of us all! We need to return to our naturalness. Each level of existence is wonderful in its own reality. It requires patience, courage and wonder to achieve awareness. Fear is the greatest enemy of humankind and needs to be faced and understood. Do not be afraid. No-one has spiritual power over another, our soul is untouchable. No-one can affect our spirit or physical by energy projection, unless we allow their energy into our space, adding to that energy by believing they can harm us. It is possible for a person to send hatred and fear energy. Some can send pictures to frighten and manipulate but these energies will be picked up by our aura and be repelled naturally if we are strong. If we are aware of choice, we can refuse to accept them. Our own fear creates more trouble for us than anyone else can.

By encouraging fear and ignorance, the few have been able to manipulate the many. The many have allowed this to happen. We have denied ourselves the right to be human in its true meaning, to reach our greatness, to experience the wonder of being part of a vast, universal pattern of interlinking energies, of which each level of existence is an important and vital part.

We are in the present to live in the present, to refine ourselves and our environment using our past-life memories, when appropriate, as experiences gained to help us; to communicate with our fellow beings, the Earth and our souls. Each day we create our future, each day should be seen as an opportunity to experience on all levels.

We can contact many levels of energy and wisdom through our own soul connection. Our soul is our connection with all others of higher energy. Our spirit connects us to our soul when we are on Earth. The chain must be kept clear to enable this communication to occur.

If we belittle and ignore our spirit, and therefore our soul, the chain of communication is weak and we feel lost and abandoned.

When we are in need of help our soul immediately senses this and attempts to give us what we need to get us out of trouble, while acknowledging the right to choose by the physical/spiritual person. This help can come through a dream, a moment of inspiration, someone may say something which sets off a train of thought, or we may open a book and find the words we need to help us. The soul tries, via the spirit, to give us a clue to help us to progress. It tunes into its spirit energy and uses all our energy centres and the brain to get the message through.

There can be a tussle between the computer-brain and the spirit energy connection as to which is the strongest at any time. Confusion can occur as the information is tossed to and fro. We then have a choice, knowingly or not.

We have many facets to our personality and we combine them all as they have to work together to achieve a completeness. If a soul needs to experience via an Earth life, the spirit energy is released with the wonder of the whole soul to support it. Our soul looks after us all the time, but it does not interfere or manipulate.

Excuses for behaviour as a physical being are not accepted by our soul when we return. Our aura record tells all and there can be no excuses or evasions. People who obey the orders of others, and use the order as an excuse for their own behaviour, are still held responsible for what they do. If we carry out an action, we are responsible.

There is no good and bad, right or wrong; there is acceptable and non-acceptable behaviour. In our life on Earth it is the choice of each person what they give into the atmosphere on whatever level. We are responsible for what we give out. We cannot pass that responsibility to someone else. Whatever we do we have to balance either here or on our return to our soul. If we really cannot do anything to rectify what we have been involved with, then we can offer help to others to help us to progress. There is no progress in feeling guilty.

Kicking ourselves mentally because we are cruel to someone does not take away the cruelty. We cannot forgive another until we are able to forgive ourselves, after doing all we can to balance and achieve understanding. To receive true forgiveness is a bonus. A person can say they forgive and still feel bitter. Until they understand our actions and themselves, and are really able to understand why we behaved in a certain way, they cannot let go. When understanding is achieved and amendment made, that is a freedom. Someone saying they forgive us, when we have done something unacceptable, may not be enough. We have to be happy with ourselves and that is what takes time, here and with our souls.

Our spirit reviews our last life in its widest sense. Our spirit on Earth has been working through an inherited physical body and the physical inheritance and experience is taken into account. Our physical body is inherited from our parents who inherited their bodies from their parents, who inherited their bodies from their parents, and so forth. We inherit many earthly things from our forebears, but our spirit is purely from our own soul. The spirit working in the inherited physical body is constantly striving to clarify and understand life, having to communicate through the physical senses to do so. It is not material success, or lack of it, that brings enlightenment, it is how we progress through care that matters. Acknowledge achievements and non-achievements, but also acknowledge trying. If we try to be responsible, and make choices, within our capabilities, that is a beginning. People can help each other, and in doing so help themselves to a greater awareness.

3
A New Life on Earth

A physical life is necessary on Earth in order to inter-relate with spirits of souls from many levels of evolvement. The Earth is the only level of existence where this great meeting of energy and experience can occur and it enables us to teach and learn from each other in a way we cannot do as souls. To experience life on Earth the soul needs a physical body for its spirit energy to reside in, to enable us all, via the shared physical body vibration, to be able to see and touch each other and therefore communicate.

When a spirit links with the physical energy created at conception, it has a memory of its soul life and where it comes from, but by the time the child is born it has lost most of this memory. The spirit, since conception, is able to travel without its physical body, linking into its energy connection with the mother and its own foetus for the energy needed. At 12/13 weeks it links to its own body completely and uses its own physical energy. It absorbs the atmosphere and circumstances of the world in which it will be living, accumulating information in order to be prepared for a physical life in its new environment. After birth, while the baby sleeps, the spirit is still able to leave the body to add to its knowledge and make contact with other spirits. It knows it cannot go back to its soul until the pre-chosen leaving time arrives, which is when we physically die. Some babies sleep for hours, some do not sleep much at all. The spirit works within the needs of its physical. The remaining soul memories are forgotten during the first few weeks of life. Babies often stare above or to the side of the head of a person who comes near during the first few weeks of life. This is because the spirit can sense the aura and assesses those nearby by observing their colours and sensing their sound. As the brain becomes active, this ability blends into the survival instinct which becomes very strong and active at all times.

The brain is a computer. It begins its programming from birth. Information via eyes, ears, nose, mouth and touch is received and processed, the baby seeking as much variety as possible from its guardians and parents, gradually building up a picture of life as a physical being. Ideally the child will be absorbed into the family and all that the family is involved in. It will then be better able to cope with all situations as it grows. A child benefits in later life from meeting all types of people. It needs to be shared to enable it to become used to the various types of people on Earth and learn, right from birth, the differences between then. If not, the child will be shocked when it has to integrate with others at a later date, when situations change or it begins its schooling. The child needs to be aware that not everyone puts them first, and learn how to deal with different reactions from people. Many children are not in an ideal situation and suffer in the hands of those who should care for them.

Children are the responsibility of their parents, guardians and all of us until they are old enough to care for themselves and be responsible for their behaviour. Adults are responsible for their own actions and for how they behave and care for those who cannot fend for themselves for any reason. We are all guardians and should take that guardianship seriously. Being a guardian does not take away responsibility from another. We are responsible for those who are unable to be responsible for their own actions. We are also responsible for how we help and treat those who, for any reason, cannot take responsibility for themselves. We are all guardians of the planet and everything on it.

BIRTH

When the day and time of our birth arrives, it is a very individual experience. On the anniversary of that day the spirit needs to acknowledge the beginning of its new physical life. Each person born affects all life on the planet. Birth is an important occasion. At our actual birth all present are affected, primarily the mother as she is the physical means of our actually being born.

The support, environment, care and love, or lack of it, have a profound effect on the mother at this time and therefore on the newly born child.

Ideally the mother should have a wonderful experience and the child should be born into love and harmony. Unfortunately the opposite can occur.

In some cases the mother does not enjoy the experience of giving birth and did not have 'a good time', was fearful, felt battered and traumatised. Some babies record this atmosphere of fear, pain, and not wanting the birth to continue as their own memory and in later life as an adult feel they did not want to be born, recalling the anguish of their mother as if it were their own. It is the condition of the mother that is recorded by the newly born child, not its own experience of pre-birth and birth. The brain begins to record after the first breath, not before. An unborn child will react, in the womb, to sound and movement, but this does not mean it is registering in a conscious way, or thinking. Physical energy changes in the mother ripple through and affect the child.

The need to honour our birth and make the anniversary a special day also acknowledges the part others took to make it possible. A great change occurs to many people when a new life begins and no parent is the same after the birth of their child, whether they see each other again or not.

The anniversary is a time to acknowledge our choice to be born and assess our progress and contribution to our existence so far. Acknowledging our parents, whatever the circumstances, acknowledges our own physical root energy and reminds us to check what we have physically inherited and change where necessary. Allowing ourselves a day each year is not taking too much time to honour life, roots and to celebrate survival and being alive. Just one day to allow ourselves to look back over the past year and tidy up.

There may be some people we feel angry or sad about, and this can be helped by communication. Perhaps we feel bitterness towards our parents, and need to take off their parent labels, using their first names for that one day. This may help us to look at them as the people they were and are, with the same inadequacies and problems as other people, sometimes unable to cope with their life.

By humanising them, we can understand more why they behaved as they did, freeing ourselves from the hurts of the past. We cannot forget, but we can absorb and detach. Some people are so personally patterned and seemingly incapable of integrating with others that they cannot reach out, even to their own children. They do not acknowledge positive life around them and therefore cannot care for themselves, and so are cruel to the weak. We do not become enlightened beings because we have become parents, immediately knowing and doing the right thing. When we have bitter memories of our childhood it is helpful to remember that hate and bitterness eat away at the person who has it. Understanding and letting go relieves it.

Humans can devalue who they are and what they have achieved themselves. They see only what went wrong, what they did not get, have or achieve. They judge themselves by achievements and happiness in others, missing their own greatness, however it has manifested.

If we feel alone and outside of life, we can help ourselves by acknowledging our own existence. If we accept our differences, instead of being afraid of each other because of our various colours, religions, sexual differences and politics, we can begin to understand, which enables us to remove our fears without losing our individuality.

Alleviation of suffering, whatever form it takes, is worth all the time and effort we have. There is no abnormality in the world, only the lack of understanding of the normal. During our new life on Earth we need to communicate and be aware of the energy sounds and senses of others.

ASTROLOGY

When our soul decides to experience spiritual/physical life on Earth, it takes into consideration energies from other planets and stars. These affect our planet and therefore all creatures living on it. The importance of this choice varies with the reasons for coming to Earth. The conception, quickening and birth time are affected by these influences and the choice of time recognises this.

Planetary interactions affect some people more than others and the birth date and time are of great importance to the spirit of some people. The influences of these energies are chosen as part of the whole life and can be used as assets or as points of change. We all have the ability to change and use energy to allow for self-motivation.

Astrology can be used as a guide when we are choosing our goals in life. We need goals which are reachable. If we have a grand goal, it is a point to make towards, but we also need smaller ones to give us stepping stones on the way. This enables growth with striving. If we reach our main goal, it opens a new phase, a new beginning; or if not, we will have acquired a great deal of knowledge and experience through the efforts made, which can be used in many ways and become a trigger for progress in unexpected areas. There is no waste.

All things can be changed and re-used. Astrology helps us to see our potential and plan our goals.

Planetary and star signs are a human symbology to denote and make usable the different influences and for easier identification. Planets affect other planets. People are affected by their own planet. We are born when certain planetary influences are affecting the Earth and we are affected in various ways. Some people will find the time of their conception or quickening (if they were noted) would fit them far more accurately for astrological readings than the time of their birth. Spiritual energy awakening occurs at conception, quickening (at 12/13 weeks) and the first breath at birth. Each is of great importance.

Sun spots affect the Earth and therefore the people on it. Aggression and war are high on Earth when sun spots are at a high energy. When there is a solar explosion, the Earth is affected and so are we. We become careless, less attentive and therefore more liable to accidents. A good astrologer could predict these occurrences and warn us to take care of the inter-reaction by knowing the sun cycles.

As the Earth moves around the sun, it is affected by the sun's sectors of energy which have become the basis of astrology.

4
Awareness

There are many levels of consciousness and awareness which are also energies; a person can be conscious, in the sense of being aware of what is immediately obvious to them, but be totally unaware of life outside their sphere and on its many levels.

Our brain, as has already been noted, is a computer and is programmed by sight, sound, smell, taste and touch. Our spirit works through the computer-brain. The greater the width of experience and knowledge of living, on all levels of life, that the computer-brain has been able to absorb, the more useful it becomes to the spirit. The more the spirit has to work with and through, the better the quality of the whole being.

The quality and growth of the spirit cannot be judged by the present-life conditions of the physical body. Some people are mentally and physically repressed when they are young. They live in old patterns recorded by their brain since birth, not able to pin-point what is causing the present imbalance in their behaviour. A shock, trauma, new relationship or change in life conditions can all cause an altered awareness which makes them decide they want to expand, to live more fully and gain knowledge of themselves and their potential. They begin to explore what is available, sensing and seeing life differently, feeling they can contribute and have a voice.

We cannot shut down our senses; our brain records all that occurs whether we are agreeable or not. We can refuse to acknowledge life and refuse to take responsibility for what happens to us and others. We can choose to allow life to move around us, at times seeming to pick us up and throw us down at will. If we acknowledge we are part of a whole experience, we can expand, grow and consciously be aware of life.

We can contact many levels of awareness and wisdom through our own soul connection. Our soul is our link to all others of higher energy. Our spirit connects us to our soul when we are on Earth. If we seek clarity in ourselves and others, the chain will be kept clear to enable this communication to occur. As mentioned previously, if we belittle and ignore our spirit, our chain of communication is weakened; we feel lost and abandoned, seeking others to tell us what to do. Each of us has a spirit and each spirit reflects a soul. A person with a faulty brain, for any reason, still has a fully functioning spirit, and any physical disability will not detract from the spirit energy. Some people treat themselves with disrespect or are destructive to others, but their spirit will still try to connect and show care. The spirit is always connected to its soul whatever happens in its physical existence.

All people are worth helping. Nobody should be abandoned. If we are aware it is not within our capability to help a certain person, then we should not feel guilty, but help and encourage them to find someone more able who can. We cannot love everyone, or even like everyone. We are still responsible for how we treat, react to and care about all other people and for how others behave towards them. However inadequate and unacceptable as humans we may be, our souls are greater than we are. Our spirit is trying to break through the restrictions and fears of a physical life, to raise the consciousness of us all and to create an awareness of quality in life conditions.

Awareness is consciously knowing that we are more than just a physcial body-machine with a computer-brain. If we have the ability to reason, we have no excuse for inhuman behaviour. Awareness encourages thought; it enables us to choose between compassion and cruelty. Awareness shows us our choices. It is part of our inner self, our spirit. Working with our physical brain, it gives us knowledge that there *is* a choice.

We are all limitless, whatever level we have evolved to. Human beings have the capacity to be wonderful. It is awe-inspiring to realise what a spirit in a human body, linked to its soul, can achieve and yet we refuse to acknowledge or investigate our link-up to our own soul.

We also have a subconscious recording system, a storehouse of information collected but not used every day, essential for imagination to be able to expand and function. The subconscious is also where we hide the unacceptable, and where the real can become unreal.

There are some people who believe the subconscious is only a depository for monstrous things, fears and memories we do not like and are suppressing, but it stores a variety of experiences, some ugly but also some beautiful.

The brain is similar to a large cupboard with what we need every day in the front and, pushed into corners on the back shelves, the things that we rarely need, or were unable to understand when we were younger, for example exciting times and memories which could not be fitted into usual life. They sit on the back shelf, not quite reachable and then, years after the event, we can have a nightmare or a strange feeling of insecurity or fear, as something in our present life triggers the past memory. If we investigate we find we have become aware that it is exactly what we need to know now, or we are ready to understand and clarify in order to reprogramme the information with adult knowledge. By understanding as an adult, childhood fears and misunderstandings can be faced and absorbed.

All that has happened to us is a part of our complete self today. All is valid and very usable. The subconscious is not a dustbin for the unacceptable, it is part of our whole being.

Enlightenment, awareness and spiritual growth are obtainable on many levels during a physical life. Choose, question and experience each event. By accepting we are an integral part of the whole structure and pattern of life, acknowledging the role of the spirit and soul in all that we do as physical beings, we become aware of life. There are no short cuts. No-one can promise awareness or evolution of the spirit or soul to another, only share their ideas, theories and knowledge of life as they perceive it. Rites, rituals and chants can change the consciousness of the participators for better or worse, but they cannot in themselves give enlightenment.

Enlightenment is an awareness of the three levels of life; the inner knowledge that all we do affects all life and all levels of life, and an acceptance of the patterns of each level, knowing that there is nothing to fear if we are aware, but that all must be acknowledged and dealt with. This is achieved individually and collectively working among others, sharing, caring and being aware of the essence of all life. Life is simple and wonderful when responsibility is taken for all actions.

When a statement is hard to understand, it does not automatically make it profound. Profundity means depth of thought, not impossibility of understanding. Wrapping a theory or idea in words, rites and rituals does not make it profound or a truth. Truth comes in many forms, but it is always clear and understandable. Many people cannot face and cope with the nudity of truth and its simplicity and so cover it with their own fears until it is unseeable and unapproachable. They seek, find and attract others to form a group. The label of teacher, leader, prophet, master, is given and accepted, based not on profound thought, care and wisdom, but on ego and need. This person is fed energy and adulation in return for a promise of progress which is not theirs to give. No person has power over others, unless that power is given to them by other people. No person can control others unless they allow them to do so. Enlightenment and awareness do not need worship and show, but inner peace and harmony.

Be aware that you can change your life, prune away confusion, acknowledge your individuality and find your own wisdom. You may not always like the clarity and self-awareness it brings, but you will be in your own light, not in the shadow of someone else. Truth is not realised through intellect; it is felt or sensed.

A wise person is serene and light because they have discovered the simplicity of life, not because they have solved its complexity. Life is simple, which does not mean it is easy.

5
Responsibility
and Care

Responsibility incorporates care. If we would give our-selves time when in a peaceful space or a pause in our rush through life to think about ourselves and our contribution, we would be taking the first steps towards being responsible people. We may find, at times, we need help or advice, but we do not learn our own strengths by using other people and their belief systems to lean on and to tell us what to do. Care on all levels is the first step to responsibility and strength, and care of what we absorb and follow is a proof of that. No truly responsible person would tell anyone else what to do, but they would help them to find their own way. We all need others, at various times in our life, but first of all we should be true to our own self on all levels of existence. Joining a society or religious group, for example, should be assessed for the strength of its ability to open minds and help its members to find their own way.

There are no chosen ones, there are no people better than others and there is not one system for all. Each person is individually a part of the whole. Our responsibility lies in how we care, what we do for others, for the planet and to refine ourselves. We are responsible for which groups we belong to, which idea of god we worship, which colours we wear and the noise we make. Responsibility is a totally personal thing. We cannot ride on the beliefs of someone else because they guarantee salvation, following them because we feel they are responsible for us, hoping that we will be among those who are saved or forgiven. There is no great puppeteer in the sky who is pulling the strings of one and not the other. We are each responsible for our actions and how others are treated and cared for by us all.

We are responsible for our own behaviour and the consequences of that behaviour and for how we interrelate with others. If a person is unable to be responsible for their actions because they are very young, mentally disabled or ill, we are all responsible for our own behaviour towards them and how they are cared for. If we know, or suspect, a child is being neglected or ill-treated, it is how we deal with that knowledge which is our responsibility. We are the guardians of all things and should take steps to carry out that guardianship responsibly.

Taking responsibility for our actions and responses in our everyday life begins a chain of energy and looking after a family is a link in the energy chain of caring for the peoples of the world. We should not undervalue our contribution. Taking responsibility for our actions improves the quality of all life and creates a tremendous energy.

In our lifetime people have taken responsibility for the care of the planet. At first, people who cared about life spoke out, making groups to protect the environment. They were ridiculed and many people laughed at them. It was hard going, but the pioneers withstood derision, sneers and insults. They gradually attracted people who had awakened to the fact that they also cared and were responsible about the future of the world and humanity. A great many were very brave in trying to stop destruction, physically placing themselves in danger, and still do.

There are now large numbers of people in all countries of the world who care and take responsibility for their input, all working in their own capacity to help. They care and feel responsible for their families, partners, friends and environment; they care when other countries are at war, about destruction and about people who are held hostage; they care about the dolphins and whales and all living creatures. Caring energy is responsible energy and is very special because it actually needs all of our levels of being, through our centre energies, to create it. It inspires, takes physical effort, gives and takes courage, uses creativity, enables progress to be made and contributes to general harmony. It is an all-embracing state of being. Care and responsibility are tremendous energies, but have to be created and fed. These energies are very strong when they combine, and like a wonderful golden essence around the Earth, they grow stronger as more and more acknowledge that we can change our contribution to the world if we all contribute to the caring, responsible energy, working towards freedom, dignity and a future for all life.

If we stop what we are doing for a moment and feel the strength of these energies within us, we will sense a wonderful pulse which makes us a part of the whole pattern of life. If we can communicate with our inner spiritual self, we will find we do feel responsibility for what we say and do; we do care about the planet; we do care about others and have already begun to listen and speak on issues affecting us all and our future. Add to that inner sense the knowledge that everything is on a lease to us, and the more responsible we become while we are here on Earth, the greater the energy of care and responsibility will be for our descendants.

The golden essence is there for us all to add to and use when necessary. We isolate and live in an unreal space when we do not care and take personal responsibility.

We are a part of the patterns of life on this planet. If we acknowledge our contribution, we will survive within those patterns.

The planet is the heart of all existence on all levels. Without the planet energy, the chain of physical, spirit and soul is weakened. Accept and understand the vast interlinking pattern of all life, instead of isolating in an uneasy importance.

6
Love and Care

The energy essence of care is a beautiful energy. It is an action energy. When care is being practised, it starts at the heart centre and spreads via our tree of life through all our centres. It is an energy which is free, it does not trap or have conditions. We can care about people, creatures, beauty, the Earth, in fact all things. We can also love someone or something with such intensity that it interferes with our progress in other areas of our life; we can worship them, carry out all their orders, do all they say without question and, because we do all this, feed their lower basic self. In that case we are not showing them care, we are encouraging them in their smallness. Caring could not accept this. Caring would involve watching their well-being, their balance, their comfort and, because we care about them, refusing to participate in or encourage mutual destruction. The emotion of love can flow freely when we care about each other. Love and care need each other for balance.

Unconditional love does not always incorporate care and can show a lack of responsibility between those concerned. Caring about a person links with love and enables us to speak clearly when we feel they are behaving in a disharmonious way and, because we care, we will want to understand. We may even feel we have to distance ourselves for a while, until understanding can be reached. Because we care, we will wait in the wings, but will not abandon them.

We have to practise detachment in order to see clearly. Some people believe we do not care if we are detached, when in fact we care very much. We detach in order to assist. Detaching in order to not get involved is totally different. That is not caring.

Love is an emotion and it can be totally accepting or selfish without understanding, which is uncaring. To say we will still love someone whatever they do does not show care but condones their behaviour. Love without care becomes possessive and self-indulgent. Every energy given generates energy. We can care and work to help people, creatures and parts of the world in need, without knowing them personally. Saying we love humankind or the world in its many manifestations, without caring enough to help where needed, is an empty statement. A stranger puts out a helping hand to someone in distress because they care about humanity, not because they love the person. Caring is a natural reaction which we all have but many suppress and others refuse to acknowledge. It shows in our everyday actions. Caring requires integration with life.

Some of us have suppressed our natural ability to reach out in a caring sense as we feel we are interfering. We wonder how others may be judging us. Some of us do not believe it is possible to care in a wonderful, embracing natural way and need help to acknowledge and experience it. Each person needs to reach out in their own way. To care we have to sense other life. If we shut out the right of others to live, we live in a vacuum of self. We need to understand ourselves, to connect with the energy of care, and then we can expand. We need firstly to acknowledge what we really are, how we carry out our responsibilities and how much we care about our own behaviour. Caring is a state of being which eventually does not require thinking about; it is action on all levels of consciousness. Love needs to go hand in hand with care.

Compassion is a branch of caring. If we care for others it does not matter if we like them or not, because we are caring on the wider scale. This is why care is so special. We can care and feel compassion for a person while knowing that they have caused their own problems. Even those whose actions we do not accept or condone can be cared for in the greater sense.

Love without care between two people is an emotional disturbance and not always beneficial. It occurs unbidden and can be impossible to stop. It does not manifest on request and can cease at any time. Love can be restrictive, obsessive and cause jealousy. It can demand change in the other person and constant reassurance.

The word 'love' is used to explain a multitude of attachments and emotions. Care is the basis of friendship. Friendship is caring for another person and not being afraid to be honest in our communication with them.

If we care for someone, we give them space, we try to understand them when they go wrong. We do not need constant reassurance. We do not need them to change to suit what we feel is right, but we can tell them what we feel.

Care has a greater depth than love. True friendship is the highest exchange between two beings. Caring in a friendship means we naturally look after the other person's well-being. We care about them even when they make fools of themselves. Love can cause embarrassment at the behaviour of a dear one. Care will overcome this and enable us not to judge.

Love by itself can become a veneer, an emotion which can turn into hate. Care cannot. Care takes time, thought and investment. It is love in its deepest, highest, widest sense. It can encompass and deal with all obstacles and does not have to be personalised to manifest itself. Care is action. We cannot care and remain passive. There are many ways we can care and all are beneficial. Each person has a capacity to care and whether it extends to one person, one country or the whole world, it is valid and contributes to the well-being of us all.

Loving someone who has become special to us and whom we care about is a wonderful freedom of expression. We can live together happily, be upset with each other on occasions, but care will make sure we look after each other through the good and bad times. Love and care towards each other means we can argue and disagree but still be concerned that our partner has a meal, has changed their wet clothes and feels 'at home'.

We love and care for our children. A child who roams from its parents and gets lost in a crowd is often shouted at when found. This is a reaction of relief from pent-up feelings of fear for their safety, and is also a sign of care. We can chastise our children when necessary and still hug them and make them feel safe and secure afterwards, because we care about their sensibilities and their need to feel accepted by us.

7
Attraction and Partnerships

Finding a partner we are able to grow and blend with through years of friendship and care is beautiful and possible. The changing times can be weathered and the connections strengthened and mellowed as time passes, moving from passion and need to joy at being together, mellowing in the glow which others recognise and yearn for; all this is possible. Many do achieve this. Others meet someone who seems so right that they give themselves totally, dreaming of many years together in security and harmony – and then feel let down and rejected when it all goes dreadfully wrong.

Why do we attract people who turn out to be so wrong for us, when we initially seemed to connect on all levels of being, and briefly life seemed perfect? We can begin a so-called meaningful relationship, but eventually ask ourselves: 'Where is that meaning now?' Living together becomes impossible and yet the thought of parting leaves such a void we cling on through pain, disillusionment and loss of purpose and dignity. Some look inside themselves to find reasons and help, trying to hold on to what was, searching mind and heart for reasons and staying through fear of being alone, eventually leaving, or being left, pining in all energy centres for years.

Our aura is the sensor which constantly reaches out to see if others are safe or harmful. We can feel wonderful next to one person and ill-at-ease or afraid near another. Some people are aura-compatible at first and can live together very well, but if they do not both acknowledge that it is vital to change and grow together as individuals, they will constantly have to compromise to continue as partners.

Physical attraction can be the first connection and if it is then backed by personality and inner compatibility, it becomes part of the whole process and works well, but some people have a need to be with and seen with someone who is attractive, whom others admire and want. Some people envy others who have an attractive partner, refusing to make contact with anyone who is not attractive. The need to be with a person who outshines them in this way can be caused by non-acknowledgement of self.

It could be personality that draws us together. A seemingly integrated person with many friends, always with something to say, always busy, can attract a quiet, reserved being and both feel whole by sharing their different energies. This sharing can last for years. Should the balance change, perhaps by the quiet partner gaining confidence and blossoming, the connection can be broken, the balance destroyed. The brightness in one partner may become calm and no longer seek light and friends and this may change the balance. The opposites become more the same. This change can be absorbed by some and the partnership continue, but in other cases one of them will be attracted to their opposite again and seek a new partner.

When a partnership has lasted over years, we can forget to show kindness to each other; forget that verbal communication is essential, expecting each other to 'know' what is wrong without speaking. The longer we live with another person, the more we need to communicate and share. We cannot remain the same all our life. When we first meet we are alert and absorbed in our new love, we have a knowingness about their needs; but as time passes our non verbal connection can lessen, the knowingness fading as life and everyday existence demand our attention.

It is possible to feel physical pain, nausea and despair when we are parted from our chosen one. This is a physical reaction caused by the disconnection of aura energies, as well as the physical removal of touch.

At times we may feel an attraction to be so strong that we cannot accept that the energy and magnetism we feel can be generated solely from ourselves. We seek reasons for the deep connection, even believing it is pre-planned, or a past-life repeat.

SPIRIT CONNECTION

We can meet a person already known to our spirit. When we sleep, our spirit reaches out to others and forms connections. A harmony can be achieved between the two spirits over a period of time. When the physical beings eventually meet, they will feel an instant knowing of each other, wondering at their similar thoughts and ideas, even sharing a love of place, similar music and literature, yet they have never physically met before. They form a partnership based on their similarities, ignoring or hoping to change the incompatibilities. The good times are wonderful, the 'knowingness' over-riding irritations. When the glow fades and they react as physical beings, they cannot connect. They become moody, dissatisfied, and begin to acknowledge that they have different tastes and needs which require attention. But the friendship of their spirits will continue, even though the connection of their physical existence becomes more and more disharmonious. When they finally part, exhausted and confused, they wonder where the magic has gone, never forgetting each other, even trying over and over again to 'make a go of it'. In some cases, after parting, the sharing and growth is acknowledged and remembered in its beauty. An acknowledgement of being friends apart is preferred to destroying each other by staying together as partners.

Those who feel that this connection is too strong to be only a physical attraction believe they were meant to be together whatever happens. They have heard or been told we all have soul-mates, a someone for each of us, pre-chosen. They believe, in spite of all that happens to them as humans together, they must never part. 'How could it be wrong?' they ask, 'we have such a strong pull toward each other.' If they find a level of harmony they could stay together, but if they stay only because they feel they should, when the relationship is floundering, they will not seek reasons and try to balance.

Our partner on Earth is rarely chosen before we are born, though souls and therefore our spirits can know each other. The spirit which resides in our physical body can reach out and find that connection, but our reason for being on Earth is to learn about each other on all levels of life. We are each an individual with our own mixture of energy levels, all teaching and learning from each other. If our partner on Earth was chosen for us, this would exclude our choice, as we are now, inhibiting growth and expansion on all levels of existence.

Our souls can certainly be in harmony and our spirits can know of each other, but it does not follow that our physical attributes, which have been copied, inherited and absorbed since birth, via background, culture, education and genes, can blend and survive close contact.

Using past lives as a reason for the inexplicable is not an answer but an excuse. We do not meet and repeat past connections from life to life, whatever they are. We change on all levels of being each day, in this life and also from life to life.

Two physical people who knew each other in a past life could only be connected by past memories of their souls. We do not re-meet in order to adjust past miseries or inadequacies. To believe that past Earth relationships, in different bodies, time, place, culture and social systems, are so important that growth and evolvement have stood still over aeons until that connection can be made again on Earth, makes striving and expanding pointless.

If two people who had a relationship which went dreadfully wrong – in the fifteenth-century, for instance – were compelled in their present Earth life to re-live the past experiences, this would mean all others involved in that past life would have to be reborn at the same time. They would have to be drawn into the patterns of the two people as they are now, in order for them to have the stage of life reset to re-create the patterns, background and circumstances which caused distress in the past. The players would be totally different, trying to play out something long gone and placed in the realms of experience.

We are all constantly changing. In our present life we cannot go back to the school we attended when we were five years old to make amends for bad behaviour at that age. All the people and reasons have changed and moved on too. The same principle applies to past lives. Just as we cannot make time stand still in this life to enable parents, teachers and fellow pupils to come together again as they were to enable us, with our experience and knowledge of life as we are to undo our childish misdemeanours and cruelties, so past-life connections are experiences gained which are usable, not repeated but recorded as experience so we can move forward with knowledge of ourselves as we have become. To believe our past misdemeanours are so important that the progress of life is held in abeyance for our sake is an ego imbalance. We need to remember that our behaviour in our past lives has to be seen in the context of the time that it occurred, not transposed on the time we are now in. A situation cannot be repeated: the play and players have changed, and all have moved on through many lives and experiences.

Some people suffer dreadfully in a relationship because they have been told they are redressing what they had made their partner suffer in a past life long ago. Two people locked together now, based on a memory of suffering from the past, does not make for progress and enlightenment on any level.

Our physical existence is a part of our soul life. Our soul is our true self and all our past-life memories are a part of our soul. Our physical life is important, but is only a part of our true being, not all of it.

Any person who behaves in an unacceptable way to another, for whatever reason they choose to give, is responsible in the here and now for that behaviour.

There is no excuse, no reasoning which can make cruelty and suffering acceptable on any level of life, even if self-inflicted. We do not live in isolation. We all affect each other all the time.

All experiences from all Earth lives are absorbed by our soul to make the whole being, just as our experiences in this life on Earth are absorbed to make us the person we are today.

PARTNERSHIP LEASES

We each need an extension in our life to relate to and love. This can be a sameness, a challenge or an easement. Many choose another human, some choose an animal or activity to fill this need.

All partnerships are on lease. We do not own each other. Partnership leases need to be looked at, adjusted, ended or renewed, but never taken for granted. A lease involves others and must be entered into with care, acknowledging it has a beginning, a middle and eventually an ending. Both parties need tending, nourishing and space to grow in their own way, each looking at their own behaviour and being responsible for all they do. There are many people we can be attracted to at the various stages of our life, for different reasons, at different levels. Knowledge of ourselves teaches us when to renew the lease and when to change or end it.

As physical beings we are all totally different and unique just as our souls are totally different and unique. We each create our own life chain, formed from past life and present-life experiences and our chains form links in the universal chain of life. All independent, individual and part of each other, the chain of life is amazing in its diversity, subtlety and interaction, for at no time can it repeat itself.

All life is different. We may share basic characteristics and seem the same as others until communication occurs, when we find the differences. It is when we take the time to look, listen and sense that we see individuality and can marvel at it.

The sexual act is a need of the physical body to use creative energy. It is as necessary as breathing, sneezing, evacuating and making sounds. We do not have to like, love or even know anything about another person to have sex with them. Sex in this context is a pleasing of the self, an exercise to release pent-up energy which can become overpowering.

When we love and care for another person we wish to please them and delight them. We want to touch, stroke, kiss, watch them and look after their needs. This need can fluctuate, but it underlies true partnerships. When we have sex in this context it is part of making love; each person is intent on pleasing the other and so harmony is achieved.

8
Leasing and Guardianship

All things in our lives are on lease. We do not own anything. Sometimes we have a long lease with an item, event or person, sometimes a short one. We are each responsible for how all things are cared for and protected, whatever form the leasing takes. We are the guardians of all life forms.

Houses, furniture, paintings, writings and all creativity are on lease to us. Should these items become outstanding due to craftmanship or rarity, they attract guardians. The guardians are the people who inherit, buy or care for them. They do not own them, they are lease-holders.

In relationships we are on lease to each other. No person can own another, it is a mutual leasing, therefore we need to care for each other and, if the lease ends between us, each should help the other to be in their own space.

We do not own children. They are on lease to us. Children are also part of the community. If parents are unable to cope for any reason with children, then others should help. The parents should not feel shame at being unable to cope, they should feel safe in saying this is so. People do not become wise and noble because they become parents. At times we all need to help. If we understand that children are on lease to their parents and are under the guardianship of us all, we realise that we are all responsible for how they are treated. We can then help each other without the fears that outside involvement can bring.

We are the guardians of all people who cannot guard themselves, and we teach each other. We are responsible for showing children a way of doing things. They can then try their own way and learn from comparison. Take the children into parks and countryside and show them the trees, the leaves, show them the same leaves in spring, summer, autumn and winter. Show them how human life begins, develops, ages, fades and dies, by the example of nature. Show them how living things appear to die but are actually changing into another energy. This is how life is; we change constantly in every way all the time.

Children need to integrate when they are small in order to feel safe. Our responsibility is to show them care and stimulation so they realise they are a part of a whole pattern of life, ever widening as they grow to adulthood.

Animals, whether they be wild or tame, are on lease to us all, as are the plants of the Earth. We are the guardians of all things which cannot protect themselves. When we leave Earth on our dying day, it is because our lease has run out with life on Earth. We are spiritually then responsible for the condition of all things which have been part of our life while we were here. A guardian who cares will hope to leave the Earth life with good memories in the minds of others.

9
Living Inside Out

We all live outside of ourselves at times, but some people constantly live outside of themselves. These people are very seldom 'at home'. They attach to people and live through them, constantly talking about the activities of friends, living in the shadow of the sorrows and joys of others, ignoring their own existence. When a crisis comes which affects them personally, they have no inner reserves, no centre to work from and they are unable to cope. They can disintegrate and panic. Many of the people whose lives they have attached to are unable or unwilling to help them. Feeling rejected by those whom they admired, they seek help from a wider circle, going from one therapist or treatment to another, constantly looking for a solution to their problems from someone else, before they have looked at themselves and what they have and are. They blame parents, school, job, society and so on for their unhappiness while ignoring their own strengths which are unused, untapped, un-acknowledged. This is living inside out.

Some people live inside out because they have a very

low opinion of themselves. They feel everybody else is better, luckier, cleverer. They constantly down-grade themselves and eventually find it extremely difficult to live with themselves at all. They cannot exist if alone, they envy people who appear to be living a very exciting life, who have many friends around them, always going here and there. They hang around others like moths flying on the edge of the light they so desperately seek. When they are rebuffed they swallow the pain and go back for more, even making excuses for the unkindness they have received. Their own light is ignored. They are afraid to be inside themselves, unable to live in their own space, feeling inadequate and lonely without other people. This need for others can eventually cause envy and even hatred of someone who appears confident and happy, but they will still spend all their time with them, mentally criticising and brooding while doing so.

Unless we are in touch with our own life-force we cannot give. We appear to be caring because we are always there and available, but the reasons are unbalanced. We all need to acknowledge ourselves and take responsibility for our own life and how we affect others. Each of us needs to take a good look inside ourselves and learn who and what we are, acknowledging what is ours and dealing with it. We can then work to remove what is not compatible.

Look at the physical to begin with and accept or change what is seen. We can be comfortable with ourselves if we try. The prototypes other people say are the correct way to be are theirs, not ours.

We need to be brave and look inwards at our own mirror to learn to know our own self. We can start by making an assessment of how we behave in the various roles that life presents. Are we acting the part of someone else? It takes courage to accept what we are. Are we coming from our centre or are we copying someone else? Are we acting a part of tragedy or comedy because others are? Are we honest in our friendships and actions?

Everyone has a need to be in their own space and sometimes needs help to find and keep that base. A person can believe everything in their life has gone wrong by gathering in the events of others, e.g. their grandmother has broken her leg; their parents are divorcing; their neighbour has lost their job, etc. They worry and get anxious, talking about these crises as if they were their own.

They are living on the edge of the lives of others. When asked what is happening in their own life, they become puzzled and ill at ease. Some of us are never in our own physical home, we are always at the house of friends, neighbours, or going from one group to another. This is a physical sign of living inside out. Our home represents ourselves. Whatever our home is, we need to make sure it is bright, secure and safe. We should always be pleased to come back to self and home after a trip out. By being selective, choosing our company with care, our life becomes interesting, exciting, calm and in our own hands.

Each of us is a community in ourselves. We go out into the world and meet others, observing, giving, receiving and finally taking back to our base all we have gathered, to sift and assess its value, and our place in the outside world.

Living constantly outside ourselves weakens our energies. We are not part of our whole being. We eventually lose our sense of being a thinking person with our own opinions. In time, the brain cannot function sharply, our point of view belongs to others. We argue or give opinions we have heard, not thought through for ourselves.

We are unable to give our own opinions, we have forgotten how. When challenged on an opinion we have given we have no answer, no knowledge to connect with. We can then become withdrawn and stay at home and our need to be with others takes another twist. People who know us begin to feel guilty or worried at the change and ask us to visit. We do, but once there will not leave, finding excuses to stay longer. Some friends who want to be kind visit us because we tell them we are not well enough to visit or to travel.

We say we are too weak to walk. They collect us by car and take us to various places. It looks as though we are living inside because we appear brave and people are coming to us.

If we actually look at this situation, one person is getting the shopping, one is driving, another is doing the washing and so on. Really we are living on the outside, constantly wondering who is going to help, having people visit for various reasons, bringing their lives to us.

If we can admit that we have been living outside, we can begin to know ourselves and choose to make contact with our personality, abilities, warmth. Then people will contact us and welcome us, not as a duty but because they enjoy our company. They will help when we are genuinely ill or in troubled times, because they care.

Experiencing life in all its diversity requires us to live inside ourselves and reach out, not to live outside reaching out further, being afraid to come home to ourselves because we do not like the thoughts, memories or emptiness that we find. We all have various energies to use ourselves and to share with others. There is no need to hide or let fears get in the way. We become de-energised, unhappy and dejected when our happiness depends on other people.

Once we realise we are living outside too much, we can help ourselves back to base. When help is needed, instead of immediately asking someone else, we will ask ourselves first. When we have thought this out, using the right to choose, and have looked at the problem from where we were, where we are and what we need, if we still cannot solve the problem, we can then seek assistance.

We will then be in a strong position to choose the best as we are seeking from our inner self. If we immediately run to someone else, we are outside and will get a variety of advice and become muddled. Sometimes advice can cause more puzzlement than the original problem. We can get lost in the opinion of others.

To view outside issues from a detached, cool space inside ourself, even for a few minutes, is a great step in the right direction. *Breathe in as deeply as possible and as the breath is exhaled, feel the brain cool and still, the body at peace. Hold this feeling for as long as possible while breathing quietly.*

True freedom can only be experienced when we live from within, in contact with our spirit and soul.

When we decide we need outside help to assist us, we then need to seek a carer who is compatible and experienced, and able to help us free ourselves.

10
Carers and Helpers

Therapists, counsellors and carers of many kinds, are available to help others achieve self-respect and motivation. There are many problems and many different ways are needed to achieve clarity. Some people seek help to go back to when they were a child, to find a point to go forward from; some seek help to choose how to progress in the present and future; some are seeking confidence.

There are many reasons why people feel lost and alone and there are various carers whose function is to help others to become independent and strong as quickly as possible and, if necessary, give them a support system while they try to help themselves by becoming in touch with their inner strengths.

People become disturbed when their life becomes difficult to manage. They wonder where they went wrong, where they are going, seek an aim in life but cannot always tap into themselves for help. They need outside assistance to find a purpose and utilise their talents and abilities. They have lost touch with their own inner self and energy.

The work of a carer is to help people they see to feel good about themselves. If we feel good, we start to try things; if we try, whether things go well or not, we are walking forward from our own base.

Everyone has a different set of patterns to weave which can get into a muddle. When help is given to unravel the confusion, the right pattern can be seen. A person can be so used to seeing misery in life, they seek it even when life is good. They are choosing to be miserable! Some people actually seek out negativity and disharmony in life, either their own or that of others. This can be a pattern copied in childhood or due to unfulfilled expectations. It can also be used to get attention and sympathy.

People choose to behave in certain ways, but most of the time they do not realise they are choosing. A carer would look for causes in this life. We are not born full of past-life disasters to wade through. We arrive on Earth clean and clear of past lives. Some people hold on to memories from early in this life caused by lack of care, cruelty, an uninspired start, lack of education and so on. This affects their adult life and the work of the carer is to help them sift through the accumulated memories to help them to find out why the past is still affecting them so strongly in the present, and after clarifying, help them to absorb the experience with understanding.

Those who act the victim, become one. Some people are professional victims constantly relating past hurts and cruelties, some use their own childhood as excuses when their behaviour affects others, even though they are well into adulthood and responsible for themselves. They find someone to blame as a reason for their actions to relieve themselves of responsibility. A carer will help them come to terms with the past and face their behaviour patterns in the present.

Our past is our present. Our present is our future. We cannot cut slices out of our life and remove them. We cannot erase memories, but we can observe them, looking at the memory, using our years of life experience to try to understand why the people concerned behaved as they did; we can then absorb the memory with adult understanding. Healing can then take place.

Psychics are healers, some of whom use their sensing ability to find out the causes of discomfort, disease and unhappiness by tuning into an aura and sensing what is at the root of the problems. This does not make them a counsellor or therapist in the trained, accepted, sense, but their work is often called psychic counselling because the translation and help given in a psychic reading and healing session counsels others to face their problems and if necessary seek regular sessions with a trained counsellor.

Unfortunately not all therapists care, and not all psychics are able to find causes. It is essential, when in need of help, that a compatible and caring person is sought to assist. Compassion and care are love in its true sense.

Sometimes all we need to help us is a lifeline. Someone trustworthy to hear our inner torments and secrets. The listeners are carers and can be a close friend or professional contact, but we must be sure we are safe with them or we add another worry to our list of problems.

11
Pupils and Teachers

We are all givers and receivers, teaching and learning from each other, knowingly or not. We show by example, we copy what we see. All that we give out, we receive. Every word and action has the energy pattern of the person involved imprinted on it.

There are many truths and theories; some theories are written as though they are truths. Some have been recorded and are believed to be truth because they have lasted for many years, their content having being squeezed and expanded into a totally different meaning.

Passing on knowledge to others is natural and progressive, but if it has been obtained from a book or from another person, we should check the source and use our own senses to feel if it is worth repeating, saying what we feel to be a truth, not what we think might or must be because someone of repute said it is so. State the source of knowledge, whether it is received from our own inner intunement or from others. The listener can then choose to go to the source if still available or question the interpretation that is given.

To have opinions we need to have experience of life on many levels in many situations. To evolve we have to be involved and to become part of what we observe. A bystander is involved in a situation because they are part of the energy of the event they are observing. Detaching and observing life gives the experience from which to voice an opinion or offer assistance. We choose to attach if we first detach.

We know what we know by the questions we can answer and should be prepared to be questioned on what we say or write. If we cannot answer, for whatever reason, we should honestly say so. The questioner and informant can then each seek the answer elsewhere, learning from searching, and from each other, when answers have been discovered.

If each person could answer honestly: 'I do not know' without feeling ashamed, we would all begin to listen and learn. We all cause ripples on the combined energy and these ripples affect not only us but all life.

Souls are also givers and receivers from the outer levels to those nearer the Earth. Each teaches by example, caring and experience. On Earth, our spirit as an extension of our soul continues this exchange. When we observe our everyday activities, we can sometimes see where we learn and where we teach, but it is a natural ongoing activity which occurs in spite of us.

Being human is a very interesting, exciting and sometimes a hard and dangerous adventure. The only time our soul, via its spirit energy in the human body, can be among other soul energies from all levels of involvement is via its spirit energy during a life on Earth. As a soul we exist mainly with others of similar vibration, although some souls do visit or spend time on a different vibration to their own in order to teach and exchange knowledge. On Earth, spirit energies from all levels of soul evolvement can be together because the spirit is housed and energised by the physical body which is the same vibration for all.

This is why we sometimes feel alien and out of harmony, on a spiritual level, despairing of others and their behaviour or they despairing of ours. Our souls come from different places. With some people we feel very harmonious; this is because their aura reflects a spirit energy which is compatible with our own.

In order to learn and teach, our soul chooses the Earth experience, via its spirit energy, as it is able then to incorporate abrasion and harmony, giving and receiving, as an ongoing and very intense experience. Via the spirit in the physical, the soul is able to meet and mix in many situations, finding strengths and weaknesses by exchanging and participating in various experiences. By doing this we extend knowledge of each other as humans, spirits and souls. The spirit energy of the planet is affected by us all. The common consciousness of humankind is downgraded or uplifted by the sharing and experience to which we all contribute and emit into the atmosphere. Life is ongoing. We come to Earth as a part of that process, not as the process.

12
Freedom

Freedom has many meanings and each person has their own idea of what freedom is. Some countries are proud that their people have freedom of speech, but that freedom can be limited by prejudice. We can be free to go where we choose but are halted by barbed wire, notices and fences.

Having money to spend gives freedom from want, but the money has to be earned or given. We can feel we are free and have all we need, happy to pay the price for our chosen freedom.

Not having material wealth and choosing to rely on the generosity of others to supply what is needed would seem like freedom to some. The fact they may be hungry or homeless does not detract from their sense of being free.

One person's idea of freedom could seem like a nightmare to another. Feeling trapped in a lifestyle, when the circumstances are opposite to what is needed by that person, is really a nightmare. Waking each morning to face another day which has to be lived through in an alien environment, with incompatible people, causes despair and depression. Freedom seems far away.

There is no true freedom where there are strings, commitments and prices to be paid, but many choose to accept as freedom what their way of life gives them.

Freedom is of the mind. The ability to think as we choose. Even though our thoughts are based on what we have heard, read, been told, seen or experienced through others, we are able to think as we choose. The wider the knowledge and experience we have acquired through listening, debating and living with others, the more freely we can think.

Freedom is not a physical state, it is a sense. If we feel free, then we are. It is a state of being, a choice. Freedom is of the mind.

13
Ending a Physical Life

Questions are always being asked about the way we end our life; why some people die in agony, if the soul or spirit are affected by the way we die and what happens to people who kill themselves.

Our soul chose, before our life began, in what period of time it wanted its spirit energy to return to itself. We cannot die before or after that period arrives. The choice of physical dying time incorporates the type of body, physical inheritance, possible life patterns which are available and the background of the parents.

We cannot shorten our stay on Earth because life is hard and unbearable, just as there is no way we can extend our stay because we are having a good time! All of us need care, love and dignity while we are living and when we are dying. Care and healing should be available to all so that they live to their last moment in peace and harmony

Our soul does not pre-choose how we die. The way we die is based on the way we live. We are the product of our own polluted society. If we take care how we live and behave, then our ways of dying will be less polluted and consequently less painful. The natural way for a person to die is by the body switching out at the chosen time, like going to sleep. It is very moving to see someone who has died this way, a person who did not wake up from sleep or who sat in their favourite armchair, sighed and left.

We need to die in order to get a new, updated body when our soul next chooses to incorporate its spirit energy in a life on Earth.

If we kept the same bodies and lived forever in them, there would be no way of refining the physical state. By combating disease and disability in this life, the inherited physical of our next life will be upgraded. The cycle of life on Earth includes the refinement of the soul through the refinement of the spirit and the physical. If we can fine-tune our physical bodies while on Earth, our spirit has the best quality material to work through. When our bodies are well, harmonious and cared about, our brain, the computer, can use minimum energy on maintenance. The spirit can then use the energy which is released and available. Equal time is needed to develop our physical and spiritual selves. One level of existence will not grow more by ignoring the other. They need each other in the best condition that can be achieved.

Irrespective of how we die, we return to our soul for integration and understanding. Certain memories fade very quickly including the pain and method of dying.

How we die is important to those still alive on Earth. People who kill themselves have a deep effect on many people which is quite different from the effect of a death through illness, accident or old age. How a person dies affects those close to the person as well as others not directly connected but involved in care. The ripples from a suicide are very widespread. People are deeply shocked and many take stock and think about their responsibility to that person. Some feel relief, some guilt, some feel sad and wish they had been nearby to help the person. Everyone concerned has a great deal of inner searching to do when a person kills themselves.

However we die, we affect our family, friends, the planet, our society and all in it. The spirit of the one who has died is free. It may be concerned how the way of dying affects others, but the spirit is complete and well.

Life is precious. Look around and try to sense those in deep trouble to offer care before they despair.

Some people get upset when they have been sitting for a very long time with a person who is ill and, when they leave the room or turn away for a moment, death occurs. When the watcher realises this has happened, they may feel upset, cheated or guilty because they had left their post at the final moment. A spirit waiting to leave the physical leaves when the person is absent, because the energy of the person on watch has been removed. Some spirits prefer to leave when their physical body is alone.

Intense physical energy near a dying person can replenish the electro-magnetic vibration of the physical body, making leaving harder for the spirit. The spirit would leave eventually, of course, but it is sometimes easier if we do not wait too intensely.

Be with them, hold their hand, but do not hover and intensely watch. Be an observer and carer. It is easier for all concerned.

No one dies on their own. All spirits are met when the dying time comes and the spirit will see those energies and reach out to them. Death is an experience for the living; the spirit is free and ready to return to its soul.

We do not die alone because our leaving time is known to our soul and our soul knows our living friends and who has preceded us. At least one spirit of a person we would recognise as having lived with us in this life, and who has already died, will come to meet us, as well as spirits of living friends who are asleep. Our soul also sends helpers to meet us and take our spirit back to its care.

Very ill and old people who are drawing near their leaving time often sense these energies and say they can see their dear friends, family or partners, in the room. Some of these visitors may have died many years before, but the spirit is able to see these energies when it gets near the end of its physical life. Some spirit energies arrive before the actual dying day so the person can get used to them and, when the time comes to leave, there is no fear, only a continuance.

The spirit leaves when its time on Earth runs out. The body then dies. The body cannot die until the spirit leaves. A machine can keep the body functioning, but when the time for the spirit to leave arrives it cannot stay. When this happens the body functions as an extension of the machine, not as a living person. If the machine is switched off and the spirit is still with the body, it will continue to live without the machine, until the dying time arrives. Life support machines enable the physical body to function and remain usable until it can maintain itself. If a spirit still has time left on Earth after the machine is switched off, its physical body will be in a better condition having been maintained by the machine and skills of carers, but nothing can extend life – such aids can only help make life more bearable.

Part II

Energy

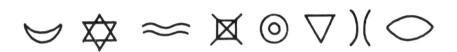

14
Soul Sound Energy

We each have a different sound and during our life on Earth we constantly tune into that sound. The energy of the sound comes from our soul, is represented in our spirit and links with sounds from our physical inheritance. However, our soul sound is our true energy and supersedes the physical sounds. It is the soul sound which keeps us moving, searching and sensing there is something greater than ourselves. While on Earth our survival instinct uses our combined sound patterns to keep us safe.

We need movement to create rhythm on all three levels of existence in order to keep our sound connection clear. We walk when we are nervous, we think better when moving, we are inspired and emotionally moved by new sights and sounds. We become de-energised and fearful when we become attached to material possessions and people; we cannot sense our own sound. The more attached we become, the greater the fear of loss and inability to cope with the challenge of life. Eventually we become the sound of what we possess, losing connection with our own soul sound and therefore losing connection with ourselves.

We need to sense our sound pattern in our everyday habits, when we eat, when we sleep, when we work and play. When our rhythm is found, it enables our physical and spiritual energy to flow unrestricted by erratic patterns. A person who does not have rhythm in their living habits becomes de-energised, muddled and physically unwell.

Society suggests that unless we stay in one place we cannot accumulate, interrelate and feel safe. Our survival instinct tells us that if we do accumulate and stay in one place we will lose our rhythm and become sitting targets.

When we go on holiday to free ourselves from the pressures of work and home patterns which are unnatural and claustrophobic, we keep a line of sound attached to our home and possessions all the time we are away, because we fear the loss of our security.

We are constantly fighting within ourselves to balance the different levels of sound.

Should we acknowledge that we have chosen to stay in one place or type of work, or have chosen to move from place to place, we can calm the internal battle and create harmony in our sound lines.

When a child cries, it is pacified by being carried by a person it knows and who is moving in a rhythmic way. The child screams because its spirit has to protect its physical body and cannot move itself out of danger, and, when it cannot see or sense a safe human nearby, its spirit causes it to scream to bring help back to its side. All the reality of life around it is recorded, often in a distorted manner, and can be sensed as dangerous, with attack possible. Life is sensed out of perspective by the unprogrammed child brain. If the screams of a child are ignored, it will eventually sleep from exhaustion or become completely silent and watchful, tuning into its own sound. Survival of the physical body is of utmost priority to the spirit.

Old people who are physically unable to move quickly will feel vulnerable and make a noise until a safe person is near. Those who are senile shout and bang objects when frightened by new faces to frighten the danger away. If the face of their carer is seeable, they will be peaceful. If not, and their cries are not answered, they will, like children, sink into silence or sleep.

When we are young, our physical and spiritual sound inheritance unites in the need to have certain patterns of sound sameness with others, in order to feel safe and secure. One of these is the need of the child to have family groups in order to know its survival is covered should the parents leave for any reason. They also sense the need for siblings, but this need can change at various times, as the reality of another child in the family interferes with their survival need to have their 'own' group of adults with a similar sound on call to themselves at danger times. A sibling could interfere with this instant response. A young person being removed from its family can defend and refuse to accuse the abuser in order to stay with the sound energy it knows, even if that means continued cruelty or danger. The sound energy they link to is preferable to the unknown sound of strangers which can be sensed as more frightening than the cruelty or danger from known sound extensions of themselves. The physical sound line between families may not be in harmony, but it has a definite similar undertone. A change of adults brings in a new sound with no familiar rhythm to the child and therefore appears dangerous. When circumstances cause partings and changes in family connections, the memory of the original physical sound lingers through life and, at certain times, however pleasant the new family may be, the adult will seek and pine for the sound line which is missing from their life. They feel the need to know and see where they were born, to seek birth parents when they have lost touch or been adopted. When the meeting occurs the sound line will be strong and familiar, and they enfold their 'lost' sound into their life. This movement enables us to go full circle and touch our roots in order to move on with knowledge of our own sound of life and spirit, which enables us to know ourselves.

Some children behave very badly to their foster or adopted family to test them for strength of sound and the extent of their care in disharmonious circumstances. This is the survival instinct activated by the physical and spiritual need to see how safe they will be in the new sound energy.

Many children who are sent to boarding school at a very young age are terrified when they arrive because their sound link to their parents has been removed. They take a great deal of time trying to find safe sound lines in others at the school to attach to. They become attached to teachers and older children in a desperate attempt to feel safe. Survival instinct is high. Some never find a safe sound and are affected well into adulthood by loss of confidence and insecurity. The longer the child is away from its parents, the more it seeks a safe sound. When children grow older, they seem unconnected to their parents. It helps children at boarding school if they see their parents often to reconnect and feel that their inherited sound is safe.

At times we can feel out of tune with our true parents and wonder if we are adopted because we feel so out of harmony. This is caused by the spirit energy having to adjust as its body grows to the physical sound energy it is living with. Each member of a family has a similar, but not identical physical sound. Some harmonise very well, but in some cases the effort needed to remain compatible with parents, siblings and relations in later life causes great strain.

OUR OWN SOUND

When we are young we have a strong connection with those who share the inherited family sound, and need to see and touch our roots of family and place. We also have a spiritual need when we reach maturity to leave the family in order to find and consolidate our own sound; we need to hear ourselves, our own harmony. Eventually we may create a family from ourselves and the sound we have, which incorporates physical inheritance as well as our own individual soul sound. A new circle begins that is linked into all past recordings. A new sound is added to the ongoing song of our life.

We need to know from whom we physically come in order to free ourselves spiritually. We are born with many physical and spiritual energy lines which reach out at all times seeking fulfilment, affecting all around us. Our energy lines are with us throughout our life and need pattern and movement in rhythm, to sense what is best for us as a total being, as we move through life. We change all the time, accumulating knowledge and information, unable to go backwards or sideways as we cannot stay the same person even if we wished to. Every word we hear, every book we read, every person we meet affects our sound energy and, subtly or obviously, changes us. Our present and past lives cannot be repeated. We are not able to go back and change any part of the ongoing sound of our three levels of life. We absorb what occurs and use it, knowingly or not.

We are not able to remove the sound patterns of our actions in our past, but carry them in our aura as part of our song of life, often unbeknown to our physical selves, but very known to our spirit and soul.

All over the planet for all times we have made and shared sound energies. They are part of the air around us, vibrating and changing us all, as we affect each other by our actions. We cannot recall and alter sounds we have emitted. We can send sound energy to try and balance the sounds we have made, but cannot hide them.

We dance continuously during our life. When we are angry we dance in a fury, when we are happy we dance with joy. Through the ages dancing has been an essential part of progress, and enhanced our ability to remember our history and culture. Dances for change of seasons, birth, adulthood, marriage and death; dances for celebration, for comfort, for harmony. Some dances have become traditional, others are spontaneous, some are individual, others are collective.

Young people need movement. They create dances incorporating the sound of youth. They move in packs from place to place, pacing out a dance, trying to frighten other people. This is their way of finding a sound line of their own as they move nearer to adulthood. They become hunters as their survival instinct tests their strengths and weaknesses. When it is possible for a young adult to experience a walk through life by travellng alone, meeting and parting from others, living with their own sound and survival instinct, they use their energy to stay alive. They become part of their own song, no longer able to rely on family to protect them, and in touch with their own inner survival sense.

Through our life there are occasions when, as we gather with those of like mind or ideas, we have found a similar sound. We may not like all our companions, but feel stronger when we blend and present a similar sound to those whom we see as outsiders.

All of us, at times, unite with others as a pack, when we sense the sound of danger. We all have a tendency to fear the loners or those who seem different. We do not like their sound. When we sense this difference we gather together to increase our own sound and energy. Anyone who does not fit our sound is sensed as a potential enemy and is hounded out. Not always obviously, but often by silent disapproval. In home areas, offices and work places people are teased, harassed and often begin to doubt themselves. Harassment is hunting to eliminate and remove and is just as violent as physical attack. The different sounds of others, whether it be their politics, religion, colour, or individual thinking are frightening to those who have chosen to repel all differences around them. They live in unchangeable patterns and fear. Understanding our different sound patterns removes fear and makes destruction unnecessary.

Whichever sound lines we choose to follow from the collection we inherited at birth, we record on them information for our sound energy and this sound is our history and combines with the history sounds of humankind, family, present self and descendants. Life is sound, sound affects us all. If we could recall our own sound since we arrived in this life, we would recapture the great variety of our existence so far. We seek our physical roots to find where our sound began and then travel on, adding variations to the sound in order to exist. If a human ceases to honour themselves, they no longer hear their sound and eventually lose themselves. Others cannot relate to them and finally they feel they have disappeared.

Each sound records a phase of life and projects sound lines. At times we follow the new line projected by our sound, and the line we have completed is woven in to the rhythm of the new. We cannot leave sound lines incomplete, as they weave into each other. We all weave sounds during a lifetime and eventually, when our spirit returns to its soul, all sound lines are sensed. Where the weaving of sounds is out of harmony, we connect with those we affected to clarify, balance and harmonise the whole pattern of life sound we have just completed. It then becomes part of the soul sound.

The sound line we bring with us from our soul was created and has been added to from the beginning of creation of humankind. We connect to it on Earth via our spirit which is the same energy sound as our soul, and combines with our physically inherited sounds while we are on Earth. As we travel through our life here, we always seek our own sound and need to have or make roots, in order to move away from them and feel we can safely return. We feel lost and abandoned when we lose touch with our own sound. When our spirit energy returns to its soul on our physical death, it hears its own pure soul sound as it nears its true life base. It then feels perfectly safe and at peace.

The life just completed can be likened to a colourful sound blanket, completed on the day we die. It has all the colours and sounds of our life woven into it – the story of our life woven for our soul to see and hear.

15
Energy, Humans and Earth

Prana is an energy which permeates the air around us. If we breathe deeply, calmly and purposefully, we absorb prana which enables us to become healthy, clear-thinking, strong and inspired. All energy, however created, becomes part of the energy of everything else, whether it be on Earth or in the space surrounding it. We cannot, either as individuals or a planet, isolate ourselves. We are part of the universal pattern. Prana permeates and therefore unifies all life, linking all life-forms together. If we tread on an ant, we are treading on part of ourselves as we all share the same prana energy. It is a part of life. Its quality on and around the Earth depends on our individual and collective output.

Our planet Earth is a reflection of us all. We cannot complain how the Earth behaves without observing our own behaviour. Humans are destroyers and creators. Nature is a computer which works to a pattern, programming itself at all times, incorporating the behaviour patterns of us all. It cannot stop and think. It cannot be nice to certain groups because they are involved in conservation, or are kind. If there is an earthquake, all will be affected, not just the uncaring ones. The Earth does not have a capacity to do deals with people. We are now part of the planet but the planet can exist without us; we cannot exist without it.

The universe does not need humans. We have become part of the universe and been absorbed in it, but are not essential. The universe is energy and there is life in various forms on all the planets, all very diverse. Humankind is one of these life-forms. Because a life-form can travel through space and visit Earth does not mean it is good, noble or enlightened, any more than a person from Earth who visits another planet is chosen for their compassion and harmony. We need to be careful that we see things as they are and not as we assume they should be, or believe merely because we are told.

Space does not mean empty. Energy is from vibration, and all things vibrate. The universe is full of energy in different shapes and forms, and our planetary energy affects the balance of other planets just as they all affect us.

When planets, during their journey around the sun, line up in a certain pattern, the vibrations and therefore energy created affects all the planets involved, including the Earth and all on it. When we know more about our home planet we will be able to prepare it, and ourselves, for these energy changes. Our planet is part of the patterns of the universe and it is one of many planets, each equally important in the universal pattern. We are creatures on a planet trying to reach a level of refinement and have to integrate with the planet Earth and learn its patterns in order to understand and integrate.

We are not yet fully developed beings and should strive to reach our full potential. In so doing we can add to the wonder of our planet by bringing out the wonder of ourselves. The essence of a planet is affected by the life-forms which are on it. The arid mind of humankind can create aridity on the planet. The creative mind of humankind enables growth and harmony.

GOLDEN ENERGY OF HOPE

The Earth has had a change in its energies. The change was triggered by the collective consciousness of humankind shifting and recognising that change was possible. The ripple of realisation and freedom of choice ran through many countries and people, who then felt inspired to stand together and demand dignity of life and spirit.

This golden energy of hope began in the minds and spirits of caring people many years ago. It has taken a long time to gather and collect itself. It is not a long time in the overall picture of the Earth, but it is to humans living in misery and fear.

When an energy affects many people and uplifts them, so that they seek their freedom, it is not unusual when freedom is gained to see it followed by resentment, anger and a need to settle old scores. Lifting the heavy weight of oppression and fear also releases the suppressed energy built up prior to the loss of freedom. This will clear and change when we all strive to understand and become caring guardians for each other.

The golden energy has circled the world and affected all of us. We have a choice in our life to look at our own selves and our fears, lost hopes and aspirations which we have suppressed, and honestly deal with them.

Ideas and theories which suited the needs of communities in the near and far past are no longer necessarily relevant. We should not confuse age with wisdom or 'new' with progress. All information and beliefs we have inherited need to be checked, taking into account where they began, their strengths in the present and ability to travel forward.

The planet Earth has three stages of life, a physical, a spirit and a soul, just as we do. We renew our body each time we return to a new physical life. The planet also renews its physical by change of climate, movement of land mass, change in water levels. It has also been bombarded, misused and polluted by humankind and we, being a part of Earth, now share the results of that misuse and are polluted ourselves.

The Earth is a reflection of the humans that live on it. When there is a great deal of anger and resentment which leads to wars, cruelties and deprivation, the Earth will pick up this energy and use it in harness with similar energies of its own. For instance, enough fire-power, shelling, bombing and burning will create energy which activates volcanoes. When people decimate themselves, mutilate each other and cut themselves off from their source, it causes the Earth to tear itself apart, earthquakes occur and the land splits in two. While people have arid thoughts, lack of care and kindness and do not send nourishment to each other, so the waters will dry up on the land, the earth will turn to dust and no food will grow to nourish us. We affect the Earth and the Earth affects us, When we change our ways, the Earth will be able to change its ways.

When our spirit arrives on Earth to experience a physical life, one of its reasons for being here is to work, via the physical, at keeping ourselves and the planet clean, free-flowing and healthy, to blend with natural patterns, correct past damages and repair as we progress. Our combined output is the mind of the planet. The planet is only as wise and harmonious as the beings who live on it. Earth is not female or male, but it is living matter and combines male and female energy, absorbing the energies of us all and behaving accordingly.

It is essential that all damage which occurs to the planet, to all life on it, is repaired and harmonised immediately it occurs, blemishes smoothed and all changes and constructions blended with natural movements and contours. Periods of rest, overhaul and cleaning of life and planet are essential.

A balanced human will blend individually and integrally with a balanced planet and both will survive as part of the universal pattern. When humankind is unbalanced, so is the planet. They then destroy each other.

The computer-like tendencies of nature will constantly try to overcome or remove any disability or handicap on the Earth, whatever it is, just as the human computer-brain strives to remove, adjust and absorb to keep the human physical functioning.

Humankind could integrate with care instead of recording itself on the energy of Earth as a scourge, illness or disease which needs to be removed. This record causes us to be shaken, baked, frozen, starved and dried out of existence.

16
Exchange of Energy

All life vibrates and creates its own energy patterns. These patterns are around us all the time and on occasions we can sense them, especially those from other people. Our aura will naturally repel any energy which is felt as alien or out of harmony with itself. On occasions, however, the alien energy is able to filter through the aura to the electro-magnetic layer and remain there, causing us distress and mood changes. This can only occur if we are disharmonised through fear, illness, unacceptable environment, the company we keep and the content of what we see and hear. Aura clearing is used to clear this, and attending to the cause.

All gifts given to us can be accepted, refused, returned or passed on to someone else; so it is with energy. Energy knowingly exchanged should be assessed as soon as it is sensed and before it is accepted as inevitable. Energy sensed which is unwelcome can be neutralised or deflected.

Energy neutralises when it leaves a person unless there is someone very close or it is accepted by someone else.

Healers prefer to work with their patients in privacy and avoid waving their hands in the air during healing because, when this happens, the atmosphere or other people nearby can be affected by the energy being cleared, as it could stay in the room or reach the aura of someone else before neutralising. Healers always discharge energy to the Earth by pointing their hands downwards when transferring healing energy.

The human brain is quite capable of transmitting patterns to another person, knowingly or not. This human ability to send and receive is common to us all, and at some time we are all able to 'know' who is going to be on the telephone, or going to knock at the door. This is not being psychic; it is a natural ability to send out energy and receive it, stronger with some people than with others.

We all share the air waves, we are all connected to each other by the vast common consciousness around us. Our ability to send and receive from one person among all others seems impossible, but we can and do transmit and receive on occasions. We can also find ourselves singing a song which, if we turn on the radio, is being transmitted. Some people hear voices in their head which, if they tuned in the radio or TV, are part of a play or speech.

A person can enthrall with communication energy, inspiring others who are listening. Always check what has been heard, after leaving the person, as the energy used could be greater than the content. Content and choice are important and need to be assessed when we are away from the speaker. If we are at an open meeting, we have the right to question and receive answers. We can admire a good speaker for expertise but still not accept the content of the speech. By listening and questioning the beliefs of others we can find what we know and can believe ourselves. We can each learn from the other. Energy exchange through speech is essential and energy can be changed and used in many ways without suppressing it or overloading it.

We all have our own patterns and energy levels, and interchange with each other. We need other people and other people need us; we are responsible for how we use that need, how we allow ourselves to give and how we allow ourselves to receive; we have a choice. Some take and take from others, always wanting more until there is nothing left to feed on. Others give and give, to please others. Neither are balanced and in harmony. To receive we need to give, to give we have to receive. Each of us balancing the energy of others. When we have something to say, we need energy. When we are animated, the energy increases. When we are angry, we build up energy, but allow it to use us and become physically destructive. Anger does not communicate clearly. We all have the need to speak and listen and to remember that others have that need too.

ANGER ENERGY

Anger energy needs to be released, but with care. Talking to a friend or counsellor about the causes and dealing with them is a release. Triggers can be found and avoided so that in the future the energy build-up does not occur.

The energy created by anger is very destructive. Some people hold down this energy and, when it finally surfaces, it explodes totally out of proportion to the trigger that seemed to be the cause. Others suppress anger and resentment, seldom releasing it. This makes them unwell and imbalanced as it eats away at their harmony and health. Some people release their anger in small spurts, rather like a pressure-cooker letting off steam, which makes them feel better, but can be irritating and disconcerting to those who live with them. When uncontrolled anger is released, it shocks and causes fear in others as the energy goes through their aura, whether they are the cause or not. It also damages the sender, even though they say they feel better to release it in this manner.

Uncontrolled energy and destructive energy affects its creators. The energy behind anger is colossal, as it is for hatred. They boil and burn, smoulder and erode, and undermine the physical being and harmony of the spirit, causing great stress. Every energy we use we have to create; we make it, it is ours. If we send out love energy, we have created love to send out and therefore become love itself. If we send out hatred, we have had to create hatred energy, therefore we destroy ourselves. Anger and hatred energy have to be fed and nurtured and eventually consume their creator.

To punch, kick or otherwise mutilate a cushion or object to release anger is a very misunderstood practice. Any one who transfers intense energy to an object can connect with the person the object represents, knowingly or not. Releasing anger in this way does not find and solve the cause which could be rooted in the person beating the cushion.

We give and receive energy unknowingly all the time. For instance, if a person helps another as a duty and not willingly, they build inner resentment, and resentment is energy. The recipient of the resentment energy will feel upset and angry, even though the resentment is well hidden. They will become difficult and unhelpful, which in turn affects the unwilling helper and makes them feel more resentful. The energy will now have formed a circle of negativity between them, resentment breeding resentment. A total change of attitude is needed to break this circle. Understanding and communication will help. Energy is sensed as it is, not as we pretend it to be.

UNWANTED ENERGY

It is essential to become physically and mentally active when we receive unwanted energy, and not become a sitting target, thinking and worrying, which allows the energy to stay and affect us.

The energy behind spells and curses is usually sent via thought-forms, or using an object to represent the receiver. In some societies they elect a special person to send spells or curses where needed, who becomes adept in transferring energy to others for specific results. Letting the chosen receivers know in advance begins the fear energy, and so an object is usually left near the person to make the intention known, which enhances the effect. When the sign is found or the energy sensed, the recipient becomes afraid, believing they have no choice, and adds this energy to that being sent. Accepting they are cursed or have a spell on them, believing they have no choice, means that all happenings, large or small, which they would usually ignore or reason away, are blamed on the spell or curse, whether the energy sent is causing these things to happen or not.

Feeling hatred or anger about another person does not necessarily mean that negative energy leaves the sender or reaches the receiver, but this can happen. When a person is frightened, they become careless and hypersensitive, and so are more likely to be involved in accidents or notice ordinary incidents and make them abnormal, blaming all on outside interference. The aura needs to be cleared and physical shaking will assist this. The receiver needs to understand that they have a choice and do not have to accept and add fear to what they are experiencing. All energy can be changed and used.

We can sense the energy of fear, hate, resentment and anger on all levels of life. We do not need this disturbance and should remember we do have a choice. We can refuse to accept by not being passive but by using our own energy to motivate and activate our physical, mind and spirit. Aura clearing is essential to remove what has already intruded. We can consciously and subconsciously reflect energy back to its source if we know the sender. We can also send green and blue energy for inner and outer harmony to help the person come to terms with their own needs and imbalance.

On occasions we can send or receive the energy of love greater than can be accepted. We each have a different capacity for receiving and giving. If the person sends love energy to another which is too strong or possessive, the receiver can feel overwhelmed and trapped. It is not always possible to get the sender to understand this energy is unacceptable and we subconsciously or consciously reject it.

When this happens, send green and blue energy to ease and help them cope with their own intensity, adding pink to ease their emotions.

All energy received can be used, changed or will naturally return to its source if not accepted. All energy is neutral unless affected by humans. If it is purposely sent and accepted, knowingly or not, it becomes part of the electro-magnetic aura energy. Do not accept energy which is unwelcome.

We naturally shiver when our aura receives unwelcome energy. Shake vigorously and regularly, to remove all unwanted energy patterns.

ENERGY IN NATURE

All matter vibrates and creates energy. The energy essences of nature can affect humans so deeply that they feel a deity or spirit is present and feed the object with energy and ritual until, finally, a character or persona is created. The human energy is absorbed and becomes part of the natural essence.

The energy of mountains can be sensed by many who live nearby and can be very inspiring or frightening. Each mountain has a different energy and forms a different character, depending on the people who communicate with it. Some mountains become godlike to those who live near, who believe the mountain speaks to them. The spirit of a mountain is treated with great respect.

Water is energy. It can gently bubble as a stream or roar as it energises with other water, as a river or sea, and increases its strength. The energy of water is very varied and when it is sensed we become very moved by its beauty and fearful of its strength, changes of mood and sound. Many believe in the spirit of water and communicate with rituals and gifts to keep it happy and beneficial.

Trees have an energy, individually and combined. They are able to send a vibration to each other to prepare for change or shock. Trees also record what happens near to them. Each older tree has a different character and people believe they can see faces on them. Their energy is beneficial to all life. The spirit essence of a forest is very strong and very changeable.

All living things are affected by each other. Humans can affect the harmony of all life. When harmony is destroyed, life disintegrates. When we harmonise with life, whatever form it takes, we acknowledge we are part of the whole life pattern and contribute to the spirit of all things.

If we could understand energy in all its diversity, we would be able to use it more constructively.

When we cease being afraid of our human differences and see them as part of natural patterns, we will then hear the sounds of each other, the Earth and the universe.

17
Spirit Energy and Out-of-Body Experience

If a person is asleep, their spirit energy can leave their body. If the physical body is touched, in distress or needs to move, the spirit must return. If a person is drugged, anaesthetised, or in any other way rendered unconscious, the spirit can leave and, even though the physical body is being touched, the brain cannot activate so no call-back signal is sent to the spirit for it to return. The spirit feels free. When a person is unconscious or under anaesthetic, the spirit can hover nearby and watch the proceedings. When the person regains consciousness they can recall all that happened around their body, reporting all they saw from above, even relating what was said. If the unconscious state is prolonged, the spirit can drift further away and begin tuning into soul energy, moving towards it. It can go through various levels of soul energy, even reaching its own soul level and connecting with its own soul.

The soul, knowing it is not time for its spirit to return, will tell it to go back. We record this as a voice telling us we must return. The surgeon or attending person, realising consciousness has not returned, will use various methods to bring the patient back to consciousness, including telling them to wake up or come back. The spirit hears this and, as the brain is now also aware and sending distress signals, has to return. These experiences can be overlaid by subconscious memories or beliefs, which colour the experience and the recall, as the brain activates fully. Some people believe they have died and come back to life. If they had truly died, they could not have come back.

When we have this type of out-of-body experience, our spirit can sense what we, as physical beings, believe happens at the end of our life. We all have different ideas of what occurs at this time. Some people believe they will go to a beautiful garden when they physically die and see friends and relations waiting for them. Others have a guilty conscience, a fear of death or feel we are judged. Their spirit, retaining this belief for a while, will sense first of all what was expected from its physical beliefs.

One of the most common memories is of a tunnel with a light at the end, which the spirit wants to reach. On return to the body, the person will recall that just as they were about to reach the light, they were called back, or that they reached a wonderful place and were impelled to return.

Some of the recall is from the common consciousness we all share. There are certain images recorded around us which we link in to at certain times and it is possible to link in to the shared images of dying.

As the spirit moves further away, the preconceived ideas fade and spiritual experiences begin which are personal to us all.

When the spirit is going towards its soul, it sees brightness and light and strives to reach it, experiencing a deep sense of peace and harmony. It is a wonderful, inspiring, loving experience for the spirit to return to its soul and it does not want to come back to its physical life after this connection. However, it has to return if the ending time of its physical life has not arrived. The spirit cannot disconnect from its physical until that time arrives. Many people, after they have had the experience of being near the soul, change their whole attitude to life; become very religious, improve their way of life; discover their caring potential and ways to use it; give themselves the time and opportunity to live in a new way, or find unused creative abilities. Alternatively, they may live in the memory of the experience and lose touch with reality. Life becomes precious to some and of no meaning to others. All these memories arise from an out-of-body experience where the brain is unable to attend naturally to its physical survival. The physical body cannot move without its spirit. The spirit animates the physical.

When we sleep, our spirit can leave the body. This applies to all people. Some leave rarely, others are out a great deal. Our spirit can help others, visit friends, travel and experience. The spirit returns to its body when the physical waking time approaches, and this return, if it happens too quickly, can cause us to wake with a jump as our spirit enters and our body can move again. Some people are inspired during the early hours and while half awake see colours or faces as the spirit memories of its travels are absorbed by the brain. During our time awake we can recall an old memory of a person and when we sleep and our spirit can leave, it will follow the memory and visit the person remembered. That person can then have a dream about us. Out-of-body travel does not have to have in-depth meaning. As in our physical life, some out-of-body experiences are deep and personal and others barely remembered; some are wonderful, others are not.

Our spirit can visit hospitals and those who are afraid or ill, while our physical body sleeps. Because spirit energy can contact spirit energy, the distressed person whose spirit cannot leave feels calmer and safe after the visit. People who are ill tell how they were lonely and frightened during the night and someone came and sat with them and they felt better. They sense the visitor as real. When the nurse or carer is asked who the person was who sat with them in the night, they will tell them they have been dreaming. Most spiritual manifestations are out-of-body spirits here on Earth.

When a spirit is out of its physical body, it senses light, not darkness, even if it is black outside. The spirit does not use physical eyes and does not need light in order to see.

Physical objects seen when awake can seem very different when sensed via the spirit, out of its physical body, and relayed back to the brain, as they can appear distorted. We have a physical impression of what we look like which is different to that sensed by our spirit. When the spirit is away from its physical self it seldom sees great crowds of spirits moving about, as it can only sense spirit energy when it vibrates in the same way as, or similarly to, itself.

The memories of the out-of-body spirit can be recalled later, on waking, as a dream of a person, adventure, travel, as a deep experience or information gained. Our brain often covers the weightless memory of the spirit moving by placing an aircraft or train around the picture it has received, as that is more acceptable than a record of free flying.

While the physical body is safe, the spirit can travel anywhere in the world. It can visit those known to its physical self and the spirits of souls it knows, who are here on Earth experiencing a physical life at the same time as itself. Should anything touch, threaten or even a loud noise startle the brain and body, the spirit returns instantly to guard its physical existence.

If the spirit visits anyone sleeping whose aura record knows is not welcome because of physical connections, the spirit will be kept at a distance and if the spirit of the sleeping person is away at the time, it will be brought back to attend to the intruder.

If we are awake and moving, our spirit is in our body. We can believe, because we feel we are above or beside ourselves, that we are out of our body, but this is a state of extended consciousness. This means we have bypassed the brain and reached into our aura energy and from this level of consciousness we can observe ourselves and events as though we are detached from our body. We have total recall of all that happens because our brain is picking up all that is experienced, as it happens, in its awake state.

18
The Energy
of Numbers

Basic numerology uses two numbers. One is the addition of all the numbers in the birth date taken to the single number (e.g. if your birthday was on 25 December 1960 your 'fixed number' would be 2 + 5 + 1 + 2 + 1 + 9 + 6 + 0 = 26 = 2 + 6 = 8). This number is fixed and unchangeable because we cannot change our birth date and it is used for situations we hope will last a long time. We can change our name and therefore the number of our name is used for moving or changeable situations.

Through the ages, numerology has been confused and muddled by many different ideas and theories, using letters and numbers from different systems and mixing them in a variety of ways. Different translation methods have added to the confusion, so that now no two ways add up to the same number and result.

Quite apart from numerology, there is an ancient and at times secret knowledge of the energy of numbers.

All numbers have a vibration and therefore an energy sound of their own, irrespective of the sound we give them in our various languages. It is this energy which is important; it is the life of the number and creates its essence. The essence is the life-force of numbers.

Our energy centres react to the essence of numbers and are affected by this energy.

They are affected as follows by the use and sound of certain numbers in our daily life.

The Energy of:
Number 1 ... affects the Soul
Number 2 ... affects Courage
Number 3 ... affects Creativity and Progress
Number 4 ... affects Physical Energy
Number 5 ... affects Emotions
Number 6 (66). affects the physical three-level being
Number 7 ... affects Communication
Number 8 ... affects Inspiration
Number 9 ... affects Kundalini/Spirit Energy
Number 10 ... affects Tree of Life/Nerve Centre

Six is the number energy of uniting, whether it be a partnership or building. When the physical brain is working as a computer and is out of touch with its spirit and soul, we react without compassion and behave in a subhuman way. The number 666, which is often spoken of with fear, actually shows the non integration of the three stages of life, resulting in the lowest level of human behaviour. When the three stages of life are in harmony, the three sixes become a different vibration as they overlap:

$$6 + 6 + 6 = 18 = 9$$

Nine is the energy of our spirit essence centre also called Kundalini (see page 30), so in truth our physical is also our spiritual, joined by our soul energy, when all are in harmony and interchanging energy.

When we are in harmony in our three stages of being, soul, spirit and physical, we absorb the energy from the soul via the soul centre which, on its journey via the tree of life, connects with all centres as it travels to join with our spirit/Kundalini centre. The energy reaches into the depth and width of our aura and returns to our soul to replenish and unite, and we become *one* beautiful being instead of three separated levels.

The life-force of numbers was known and respected in the past. Buildings, such as the great temple of Jerusalem and the pyramids at Giza and elsewhere, in the world were constructed with great care and expertise using measurements specifically chosen to bring the building alive, by utilising specific number essences in the building. The great temples and pyramids always had the most knowledgeable and experienced masons, architects and mathematicians involved in their conception, building and birth. Meticulous attention was given to every detail of number energy at every stage of building, including its use and effect on humans using it. The surrounding countryside was also important and was sensed and measured out using its natural patterns, lines and water flow in order to ascertain its number energy in relation to the building being constructed. When the whole was completed the inside and outside were covered, coloured and furnished with the same care, to ensure the energies of these additions corresponded with the number energy of the whole.

If, by some catastrophe, the building was demolished, another would if possible be placed on the same site to the same specifications as soon as possible. If another temple or pyramid was needed elsewhere, the same number energy was strictly adhered to. The masons, mathematicians and architects had the secret knowledge of the life-force of numbers and therefore creation, and were held in high esteem and reverence. In later years, the alchemists sought the knowledge of the life essence through measurement of the various components of materials and spiritual energy balance. They used their own life essence from their centres to change matter, as this is also based on number energy.

Our calendar is very new compared with those of other cultures, but because so many use its number energy, it has taken on a life essence of its own. Great hopes and fears have been attached to the year AD 2000. The year 2000 has no meaning as far as Earth age is concerned, but because people believe it has and energise the idea, it will be special.

When we are born we are nought years old; when we reach our first birthday we have already lived a year. Our calendar is the same. When we reach the year 2000, it will be over. To use the number energy of 2000, we should begin our celebrations on 1 January 1999, culminating on 31 December 1999 as the end of the year 2000, but as we have added our energy to the energy of the number 2000, we have created a special energy.

Each year has an essence attached to its numbers.

$$1992 = 1 + 9 + 9 + 2 = 2 + 1 = 3$$

Three is the number energy which relates to creativity and progress. In its opposite, it is jealousy and envy. We had a choice in 1992 – to be creative and progress or be jealous and envious.

$$1993 = 1 + 9 + 9 + 3 = 2 + 2 = 4$$

Four is the number energy which relates to physical energy. In its opposite it is anger and resentment. We have a choice in 1993 to construct with our physical energy or destruct through our anger.

$$1994 = 1 + 9 + 9 + 4 = 2 + 3 = 5$$

Five is the number which relates to emotions. In its opposite it becomes hate and obsession. We have a choice in 1994 to love open-heartedly or destroy through hate.

$$1995 = 1 + 9 + 9 + 5 = 2 + 4 = 6$$

Six is the number of humankind. It is a very important number energy. In 1995 we will reach a stage where we can communicate as physical/spiritual beings in touch with our soul or show our unreasoning robotic nature to the world and all life on it.

$$1996 = 1 + 9 + 9 + 6 = 2 + 5 = 7$$

Seven is the number energy which connects with communication. In 1996 we can choose to communicate with ourselves and others around the world in an open and honest way, or we can individually and/or collectively shut down, refusing to communicate and therefore become isolated as individuals as well as communities.

$$1997 = 1 + 9 + 9 + 7 = 2 + 6 = 8$$

Eight is the number energy which connects with inspiration and aspiration and also contains the essence of continuance. In 1997 we can choose to use this energy to form an inspired campaign for the continuance of life on earth, or become depressed and shortsighted about the future.

$$1998 = 1 + 9 + 9 + 8 = 2 + 7 = 9$$

Nine is the number energy which connects to spiritual awareness and recognition of the soul, spirit and physical unity whilst we are on Earth. We can use this energy in 1998 to reach inwards and from our spiritual strength reach out to balance our physical life.

$$1999 = 1 + 9 + 9 + 9 = 2 + 8 = 1 + 0 = 1$$

The energy of the number one relates to the soul existence. In 1999 we can utilise this energy by acknowledging we are part of life in its greatness on Earth and, via our tree of life centre, reach up to our full potential as part of our soul energy.

$$2000 = 2$$

The energy of the number two connects to courage and security and we can utilise this energy in the year 2000 to stand strong and feel courageous about all matters connected with the quality of life for us all.

These annual number energies affect us because we have given them energy through our choice of calendar system. The more a number is used collectively and individually, the stronger its energy becomes.

19
Exercise:
Soul Connection

There are many ways to connect with our soul energy via our spirit and physical. The following exercise is one of them. The location of the centres is given in the Aura Energy section beginning on page 148.

Set a ten-minute buzz alarm. Take your time, do not expect, do not think, as this activates the imagination which can dictate or cut off the experience. Observe, sense, experience.

The exercise can be practised daily or at longer intervals. It is safe to practise this as long as you end the exercise when the chosen time arrives. Should you not stop at this time you could find hours have passed by when you do finish. This is not dangerous in itself, but shows you have missed the point of the exercise which requires you to remain aware and experience.

Sit comfortably with your hands on your lap, palms uppermost, finger and thumb on each hand making a circle.

Breathe and connect with each centre: breathe in, feeling the breath going through the golden soul centre (at the top of your head) which shares space with inspiration; breathe out to the communication centre (around the lower part of the head and neck).

Breathe in through communication, inspiration, and soul centre, and out to emotion. (The emotion centre lies between the top of the shoulders and the middle of the ribs, including the arms and hands.)

Breathe in through emotion, communication, inspiration and soul centre and out to solar centre (based in the middle of the ribs down to the top of the hips) to connect with your spirit essence.

Breathe in from solar centre through emotion, communication, inspiration and golden soul centre, and out to creativity (based in the lower body from the top of the hips down to beneath the feet). Your spirit essence will then reach into the Kundalini centre (at the base of the spine).

Take a deep breath and feel the energies rising within you, linking each centre, as it travels via the tree of life (based in the core of our physical body, beginning above our head and finishing beneath our feet) to the golden soul centre. Breathe out sensing your energy at the top of your head. The Kundalini spirit energy is now connected via all energy levels to the golden soul centre, which is within and around the skull.

Sense the golden energy in the upper head Be a part of that energy. Be part of the true energy source. The golden soul energy may be sensed as a bowl, a saucer or a goblet. Sense the energy rising slowly as it moves into the aura, expanding and revolving in a clockwise direction Do not look for experience – it will come to you. Allow yourself to be at peace and in harmony with your whole self. You may feel you are floating or leaving your body; in reality you are expanding your consciousness. You may experience images relative to yourself now, or in past lives.

Be at one with the energy, feel it permeating your physical and spiritual self, reaching in and around you.

To end the exercise, begin at the golden soul energy above your head and breathe gently in through this centre, breathe out through communication, breathe through each centre, until you reach the creative centre and Kundalini. Breathe normally. Open your eyes, touch a solid object and move with gentleness and grace. Drink some water.

Do not spend more than 10 – 15 minutes on this exercise to begin with. If you extend the time too quickly, imagination will take over and the exercise is invalid. Lengthen the time gradually, but usually 20 minutes is found to be sufficient. This exercise calms and strengthens. We are at one with our inner self and can absorb the energy of our soul. The experience brings peace, harmony and relief from our day-to-day troubles.

Our spirit energy can link into the golden soul centre during our sleep and dreams of approaching and sometimes entering an object shaped like a giant saucer, surrounded by colour and light can occur. This can be interpreted as being on a UFO as the experience is very deep and records strongly in the brain. The experience can also record meeting figures or shapes which seem totally real in or around the saucer-shaped object. On waking, our brain is convinced that the experience has been a physical one and nervous reactions can occur, such as nerve rashes on various parts of the body.

20
Exercise: Soul Energy plus the Essences of Life

If certain natural energies are purposefully tuned into, the result can be very beautiful. A group of people is usual for the exercise, as they energise the room and can exchange experiences and senses afterwards to expand and clarify what happened for each of them.

Gather together various objects to represent the Earth and all on it. For instance:

> a ring (gold)
> a bracelet (silver)
> a selection of gem stones
> plants in earth
> flowers in water
> a piece of pottery
> shells
> crystal
> a sculpture

a fir cone
a lighted candle
models of animals, birds, fish

Sit in a circle around the objects. Do not touch each other. Choose a co-ordinator. Work through the breathing exercises as mentioned in the Soul Connection section (page 117) until the upper aura golden soul energy is reached. Sense and absorb the golden energy, harmonising and balancing yourself.

The energy can then be projected to the objects in the centre when the co-ordinator feels all are ready. The energy of each person will collect in and around the objects to form a large bowl or saucer shape in the middle of the circle. This will rotate in a clockwise direction if there is harmony, and various vibrations will be experienced by each individual, manifesting in colour, shape, smell, sound and touch. The depth of experience is personal, but the energy will reflect the level of the majority. Do not expect – just experience. After five to ten minutes the co-ordinator should ask all present to breathe gently, sensing their energy returning from the centre of the room. Each will receive their own extended energy, not that of any other participator. Breathe downwards through each centre, breathing out through the centre immediately below, as already mentioned. Open your eyes. Complete by touching a solid object and moving physically. Drink water.

The images, energy projected and combined harmony will stay and become part of the room, for all to share.

Try different combinations of objects. Experiment to find which are in harmony with each other.

21
Energy Rod

Humankind has always sought ways to heal, and various ways and devices have been invented and utilised through the ages to assist this natural ability. Combining copper with quartz is one of them, and is called an energy rod or energy wand (see opposite page).

The rod can be any size but the following is very usable:

- a piece of copper tubing approximately 12 ins (30 cm) long and ¾ inch (2 cm) in diameter;

- one, two or three pieces of white quartz of equal size, or small pieces to fill the tubing behind one large piece;

- some material to bind the tube.

Make sure the materials are clean and clear by using the cleaning method (see pages 129 – 131). If three pieces of quartz are being used, put one piece pointing outwards

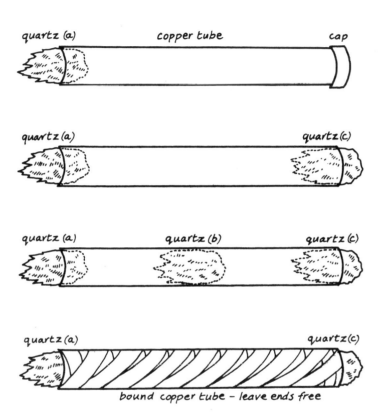

quartz (a)   copper tube   cap

quartz (a)   quartz (c)

quartz (a)   quartz (b)   quartz (c)

quartz (a)   quartz (c)

bound copper tube – leave ends free

Energy Rods

about half an inch in one end of the tube (a); push the next piece half way down the tube, pointing the same way (b); push the third piece of quartz in the end, pointing in the same way (c), protruding slightly at the base. You now have a piece of copper tubing with three pieces of quartz all pointing the same way, equally spaced, protruding at each end, firmly wedged in.

If one piece of quartz is used, it should be pointing out of the end of the tube (a) and a copper cap put on the opposite end. If two pieces of quartz are used, put one piece (a) pointing outwards, at one end of the tubing and one at the other end (c), facing the same way, protruding at both ends. Bind the tube for easy handling, leaving the top and bottom open for the quartz to extend. Hold the completed rod and direct the pointed piece of quartz at the area on the patient you feel needs healing energy. White quartz helps all centres, but different quartz can be used for specific centres.

For instance, rose quartz is very good for balancing the emotional centre, energising the arms and healing flesh wounds. Yellow quartz strengths the solar centre, mauve quartz balances communication, red quartz gives physical energy, blue quartz lifts depression and inspires, green quartz encourages creativity and progress.

A variation is a glass tube instead of copper. This can be varied in length and diameter and filled with small pieces of quartz, all of one type, or a variety. Place a copper cap at each end of the tube and point it at the person in need of healing energy. Some people attach an electric pulse to the rod to energise the quartz. Coloured glass can be used instead of quartz as the colour of the glass also has a beneficial energy.

22
Neutralising Energy

LEY LINES

Ley lines are the electro-magnetic energy of the Earth. This energy can criss-cross, spiral, bend and curve, forge in straight lines, travel across miles or cover a few yards. It covers the entire planet. Some areas have a great concentration of this energy and others have very little.

It is a natural neutral energy. It is not good or bad, male or female, it is pure energy. Humans affect ley energy and ley energy affects humans. Intense human energy will record on ley energy and its patterns will be felt by humans long after the event.

When human actions are recorded on an energy line which is dry, the record remains in the place it occurred and will gradually fade if not fed by more human interaction.

Should the ley energy be accompanied by flowing water, all actions by humans on that ley energy will be recorded and will flow with the water, affecting all who use the energy line for whatever reason, as far as the water flows.

Ley energy can spiral deep into the Earth or up and out in a large cone shape. When ley energy was respected and used with care, as at Glastonbury Tor, these immense spirals were carefully covered with earth to become man-made hills. The line of the ley energy was cut into the hill as a spiral pathway from bottom to top where a large stone with magnetic properties was placed. People who wanted to experience the life energy of the planet, to receive energy to improve their health or inspiration, would walk up the hill around the spiral path and touch the stone at the top, to give and receive as they could. Some tors were so high that small seats were cut into the hillside for climbers to rest in on the journey and, at some of the sites, food and drink were placed in these niches to refresh the climber.

Where straight ley energy lines crossed over each other, the centre point was marked by a large single magnetic stone, or each line was marked by stones making a circle which acted as a battery for the energy. People would enter the circle and when they had received the energy they needed, or instructions from the ley energy guardians, they left the circle and moved clockwise, outside the ring of stones, to replace the energy they had used.

Some ley energy zig-zags and when this energy was found by people of the far past, they covered the curving ley energy with earth to its height and walked along the top to experience the earth energy. This appears as a snake when seen from above.

Ley tors, mounds and zig-zags were built not as burial mounds, but in order that all could benefit by walking in pure energy. These sites were carefully guarded and only those who understood the importance of the energy were allowed to use them.

People, on occasions, build houses on ley energy. Whatever happens in the building is recorded on the energy and will affect certain people who stay in the building. The effect can be wonderful or depleting, nightmare creating or peace-giving, affecting health and thinking, depending on the human activities which have fed the ley line energy over time.

When it has been established that imbalance is caused by ley energy and it is adversely affecting the people in a building, the effect can be neutralised by clearing and coppering each room and, if possible, the outside as well.

Copper neutralises ley energy and copper wire is easiest to use. Cut it into pieces half an inch (1 ¼ cm) long. Each room needs to be treated.

Beginning at the doorway of each room and moving clockwise, tap a piece of copper wire into the floor, touching the wall, in all corners and projections. When the room is completely coppered, move to the next room and repeat. All landings and stairs should also be coppered in this way.

When the inside of the house has been coppered it is beneficial, if possible, to treat the outside of the house in the same way. Moving clockwise from the front door, hammer pieces of copper into the ground, touching the house at all corners and projections.

When this is completed, go inside the house and carry out the flower, candle and salt ceremony in each room (see overleaf) and around the outside of the house if possible.

Small copper objects in rooms help keep the balance. In a room which is used for healing of any kind, a lighted candle in a copper container will keep the atmosphere clear.

ROOMS

Houses and rooms are affected over years by people using them, leaving impressions in the brick and wood. Usually regular cleaning and fresh air blowing through neutralises a great deal of the old energy. However, unwanted essences can built up even from a person who is out of harmony who visits for a few hours. They too can leave an energy which can upset the atmosphere, people and animals.

When moving to a different house, clear the old energies before leaving your old house and then clear the energies left in the new house as soon as possible.

The following ceremony will enable this neutralising to occur.

Needed: flowers
            a candle and matches
            salt

To neutralise a whole house or flat, go to the room furthest from the front door. Put flowers in the centre, light the candle and place it with the flowers. With salt in the palm of your hand, go to the door and walk clockwise around the room scattering salt along the edges. When you reach the door again pick up the candle, go outside the room, shut the door and salt along the bottom of the door. Repeat in all rooms, until the front door is reached which you salt outside.

When every room has been treated return to each room, stand in the centre and fill the atmosphere with healing energy by slowly turning with hands held high. This ceremony can be carried out alone or with compatible people.

If possible, the lighted candle should be carried clockwise around the *outside* of the house, salt being sprinkled and flower petals and/or herbs scattered.

If one part of a room is affected by the energy of a visitor who has caused disharmony, salting after placing the flowers and lighted candle on the affected spot will neutralise the energy left by the person.

OBJECTS AND JEWELLERY

Humans and animals remove unwanted energy by shaking their bodies vigorously. Involuntary shivers or tremblings are the aura clearing itself.

Objects made of natural materials cannot clear themselves of past energy and over years they can collect and store not only picture impressions, but also the feelings which accompanied them, from the people who used them.

Rocks, stones, quartz, wood, metal, all absorb and store, sometimes for thousands of years. If we wear these items or have them around us without clearing the energies, we can sense and be affected by everything recorded, knowingly or not.

A piece of jewellery previously worn by another person, who had a traumatic experience or illness, can effect the well-being of the present wearer as they absorb the energies already there. Past events and feelings picked up from the article can cause the present owner to change personality or experience depressions, aches or pain totally unrelated to themselves.

Articles of clothing which have been used by another person and not been cleaned or washed can hold their vibration, which can affect a new wearer. They should therefore be thoroughly washed or cleaned before use. This will remove past energy recordings.

There is a simple and effective way of clearing past energies without removing the pictorial record of the object. Once cleared, the article will hold the energies of the present owner or user.

Only use the following cleaning method with articles which are water-resistant. For the process you will need:

a non-metal dish
a non-metal sieve, or tweezers
a piece of white cotton cloth
a piece of black cotton cloth (velvet)

Half fill the dish with water which has been boiled and allowed to cool. Place the articles in the water. Put your hands around the dish, fingers linking if possible. Gently rotate the dish anti-clockwise until the surface of the water swings to the left, sensing the past going back to the past. Pause. Rotate the dish clockwise, until the surface of the water swings to the right, feeling clean, clear colours entering the water, via your energy. Pause. Without touching the water with your hands, remove the articles from the dish. You can use household gloves, non-metal tweezers, or strain the water through a plastic sieve. The dish should not be used again until it has been thoroughly washed.

Without touching the articles with your hands, transfer them on to a piece of white cotton cloth and gently dry them with an anti-clockwise and then clockwise movement of your hand. Transfer the articles onto the black cloth and gently rub them anti-clockwise and then clockwise.

The objects are now ready for use. They will retain the pictures of their past, but not the energy holding the feelings. The objects will be clear for the new owner to record on. If you are the new owner, hold the items in your hands and fill them with your own energy. If you are clearing them for someone else, do not touch them; pass them to the new owner to hold and energise for themselves.

If the article is not waterproof,or is too big for a dish, use a blue cotton cloth anti-clockwise and clockwise instead of the water, then use the white and black cloths to complete the cleaning.

Large articles of furniture can also be cleared of their past owner vibrations. Use a blue cloth, moving the cloth to the left and then to the right, sensing the old energies leaving and the new energies entering, then rub with the white cloth, and polish with the black cloth.

When secondhand cars are cleared in this manner, be sure to clean the inside of the car, especially the driving seat. A past owner who was erratic or unsure could affect the driving of the new owner when the wheel is held and the peddles pushed.

Part III

Healing and Aura Energy

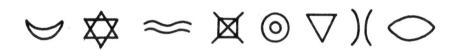

23
Using Healing Energy

All creatures are self-healing, but on occasions the energy needed to heal is not available from the self. When a person is low in energy due to illness, shock, pain, pollution or stress, they need energy to replace the loss as quickly as possible to bring back balance, strength and harmony to relieve pain and help them find a solution to the cause. When they cannot replace it themselves, a healer is able to give them the energy they need. The ability of a healer is to transmit pure energy to another person so that they can replenish and heal themselves. Healers do not heal or cure another being; they enable that being to help themselves in their own time and way.

Healers come in all shapes, sizes, colours or creeds. Irrespective of their looks, healing beliefs or lifestyle, if they care about life and the well-being of others, the energy transmitted will contain compassion and care. If the healer despises others, allows personal preferences to interfere, is self-important and uncaring, the healing energy will still flow, but the recipient will sense the lack of giving, quality and care. The benefits will be minimal.

A person in need should choose a healer they feel safe and in harmony with. All are different. Their difference is the energy which they can transmit to others.

Some healers can use their psychic sensing ability to find the cause of the energy loss, so the recipient confronts the cause and becomes as complete and well as it is possible for them to be. Some healers cannot sense or diagnose causes, but this does not mean they are less of a healer. A healer does not have to have religious beliefs, be celibate, meditative or periodically isolate from fellow beings in order to transfer the healing energy.

In fact, the greater the connection with people, the freer the thinking and the wider the experience of life, the better the quality of energy and the ability to give will be and, for those who can sense the cause, the wider the spectrum to translate from.

Healers do not need to be in a small room with chosen sounds, coloured lights or smells in order to work; they can work anywhere, in any conditions. Of course it is pleasant to have a quiet, harmonious place to work in, and this is also good for the harmony and comfort of the person in need, but it is not necessary.

When energy is transmitted from a healer to another person, it benefits the healer as well. The first wave of energy the healer receives balances and cleans them. They do not give their own energy to others. If transmitting energy physically tires the healer or de-energises them, they could be using their own physical energy which is not healing energy at all. Healers get physically tired if they work over a long period, as do all people, but not from transmitting energy. The energy flows with no effort at all.

People become unwell and uneased from a multiplicity of causes. Some people believe we are punishing ourselves when we are ill, that we do not love ourselves sufficiently, or are clearing a past-life over-shadow, but not all illnesses are self-inflicted, not all mishaps are pre-planned. We can become part of the imbalance of another person, their misjudgement or carelessness can infringe on our life, or chain of events. We should not feel guilty when we are unwell, but look for the cause, seek healing energy and move on. We are products of our lifestyle and society and are affected by it. When our physical being is polluted, its self-healing properties are weakened and we become prone to the diseases of our times. Some people say everything has a purpose and so it does, but sometimes the purpose or reason is for others and not solely for ourselves.

Sometimes a reason or a purpose needs to be found to use the period of incapacity well and a time to reflect and rest is needed and used. Past lives do not cause illnesses in the present, but a memory of a past life can be triggered when we are in certain situations. Looking at the positive outcome in all that occurs, even its effects on others who become involved, may need time, but is healing in itself and strengthens our energy field, relieving the feeling of being a victim.

All that happens around us is not always created by us as an individual. We can become part of a chain of events. Even so, we can find our strengths and weaknesses from our experience, although the trigger belonged to someone else. When we look back on a period of our life, we can often see the pattern or series of events which occurred and how we became a part of them, and then see some purpose or reason for what happened, whether we were the main player or someone else was.

A healer who cares and is able will help people to understand the reasons or purposes of what has happened to them. We can look back and find we have been through a period in our life which was very gruelling, very personal and harrowing, and we cannot see why it had to be so hard. There is absolutely no reason or purpose we can find. When this occurs, we should look to see who *else* was affecting us and who was also affected by the events at the time. Someone might need our understanding. Things which occurred will not only have affected us.

We do have a choice as to how we deal with events which occur in our life.

Note:

In my previous book *As I See It* . . . , various ways of transferring healing energy are given, including aura, touch, laser and centre balancing. The rest of this section (Chaps 24 – 28) extends the choice.

24
Projecting
Rings of Colour

A very effective use of healing energy is to project rings of colour to spin around the person in need, or around ourselves.

THREE RINGS

Breathe in through each energy centre, and out through the centre immediately below (see pages 117 – 119 on energy centres), until the creative centre is reached. Take in a large breath and, as you breathe out, feel energy rising until it is above your head. Project this energy to the person in need.

Sense three rings, one each of pink, blue and gold (or any combination sensed) spinning in a clockwise direction around the solar centre. This will keep a person in a secure and strong space when they feel threatened or afraid.

FIVE RINGS

Sense blue energy forming a clockwise spinning ring around their head, then mauve energy forming a spinning ring around their throat, a red and pink ring spinning round their heart centre; yellow spinning around the solar centre; green energy spinning around creativity and progress which includes the legs. Look away to cut the connection. The rings will spin up, down and around.

This method cleans, clears and revitalises each centre. The healer can also use this method on themselves by sensing the rings forming around their own energy centres and spinning. Some healers find looking into a mirror helps them when healing themselves in this way. Project the energy onto the reflection in the mirror which will return the energy to the sender.

25
Absent Healing

Absent healing is the sending of energy to a person who is unable, for various reasons, to visit a healer. When the healing energy is received it reacts in different ways to suit the person receiving it.

In some cases a change can be noticed immediately; in others it takes time for the benefits to be realised.

Where pain is present, many feel immediate relief which encourages them to look for the cause and correct it if necessary. However, the pain is not always where the trouble lies and the healing energy will go straight to the centre affected and begin to work on the cause. In these cases the pain may remain longer until the cause has been balanced.

If a person has created an illness for a personal need or excuse, they may refuse to feel well because their reasons for being ill have not been sorted out. The healing energy will strengthen the spirit connection and the person will feel stronger and so be more able to deal with the background problem.

26
Energy Extension

If a person is feeling overburdened, depressed, fearful, small or inadequate, different coloured gem stones or pebbles backed with healing energy will clear the aura and allow the spirit energy to extend into its own aura space. For this healing method you are advised not to use quartz as its energy can interfere with the natural aura energy of the patient. Stones and pebbles do not disturb the natural balances. The stones are used for their shape and colours and to create a pattern as the healer works. Try different kinds of stones to find the ones which feel in harmony with you. Collect about six different ones, keep them in a pouch together after cleaning them. Hold the stones in your hand in front of the person you are working with, and you will sense which one is right for them at that time. Hold the chosen stone in your cupped hands and gently breathe on it; this extends your energy to the stone so that it is a part of the healing energy.

The stone is held a minimum of six inches (15cm) away from the patient, for a few seconds. Sit the patient down, feet touching the floor, hands palm down on their lap. (See the illustrations on page 144).

1 Hold the stone in your right hand. Stand behind the person and place your hands on their shoulders, gently stroking them to tune into their rhythm and make contact. Breathe quietly, sensing the healing energy between you.

2 Holding the stone in your right hand, lift it above their head, your left hand resting on their left shoulder. The stone, plus your healing energy, will enable their natural inner spirit energy to extend in its own aura space. Allow your hand to move up and down as it finds how far their spirit energy is ready to extend at that time.

3 Stand by their right shoulder, holding the stone in your right hand, in front of their forehead, third-eye position, your other hand at an equal distance behind their head. Do not put the stone in your other hand for these two centres.

The next stages require you to change the stone from hand to hand.

4 Hold the stone in front of their throat, your other hand an equal distance away at the back of their neck, allowing your hands to move if they will. Pause. Put the stone in your other hand.

5 Hold the stone behind their neck, your other hand in front of their neck the same distance away. Pause.

6 Hold the stone behind their back, level with the heart centre, your other hand in front of their heart

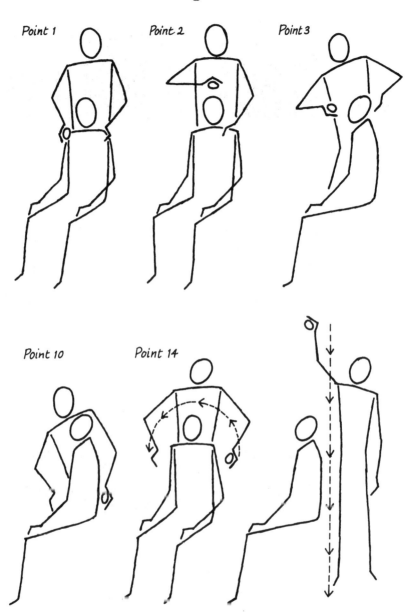

Stone Healing

centre at an equal distance. Pause. Put the stone in your other hand.

7 Hold the stone in front of their heart centre, your other hand an equal distance at the back of the heart centre. Pause.

8 Hold the stone in front of their solar centre, with your other hand an equal distance behind the solar centre. Pause. Put the stone in your other hand.

9 Hold the stone behind their back, level with the solar centre, with your other hand an equal distance away in front of the centre. Pause.

10 Hold the stone level with the base of their spine, the creative centre, with your other hand an equal distance in front of the creative centre. Pause. Put the stone in your other hand.

11 Hold the stone in front of the creative centre with your other hand an equal distance from the base of their spine. Pause.

12 Stand behind the person. Put the stone in your left hand, opposite their left temple. Pause. Put the stone in your right hand, holding it opposite their right temple, your other hand an equal distance away on the left. Pause.

13 Hold the stone at the right side of their neck, your other hand an equal distance away at their left. Pause. Put the stone in your left hand, your other hand an equal distance away on their right side. Pause.

14 Hold the stone at the heart centre level at their left, your right hand an equal distance away. Pause. Put the stone in your right hand, your left hand an equal distance away at their left side. Pause.

15 Hold the stone at their right side opposite their solar centre, your other hand an equal distance away on

their left. Pause. Put the stone in your left hand, your right hand an equal distance away on their right side. Pause.

16 Hold the stone opposite their creative centre on their left side, your right hand an equal distance away on their right side. Put the stone in your right hand, your other hand an equal distance away on their left side.

These positions should not be held for longer than a few seconds. The hands should be allowed to move towards and away from the person as the inner energy finds its own balance in the aura.

Stand behind the person and hold the stone as high above their heads as possible. Bring the stone down in a straight line behind their back and touch the floor. Repeat this action once more.

17 Put the stone down. Stand behind the person, with your hands on their shoulders. Sense the healing energy going to them and distributing through all their centres via the aura energy. Pause. Go to the front of the person and hold their hands together to symbolise that the energy is now their own.

18 Walk away from the person to give them their own space. Ask them to stretch and reach out into their own space.

The above method clears the aura, removing negative energy. It enables the person to reach out into their own aura space to replenish and sense their own courage and strength.

Do not place a stone or pebble in each hand. The rhythm created by passing the stone from hand to hand is very important. Each stone and pebble have different qualities. No two stones or pebbles could be exactly the same even if split in two.

When the person has left, hold the stone and feel it clearing. Put it back with the others in its pouch until needed again. Do not let anyone touch the stone. If they do, clear it immediately under running water before replacing it in the pouch.

27
Aura Energy

There are many questions relating to the aura, including what it is, what it does, how it affects us and why so many explanations are at variance with each other. The aura has been spoken and written about in various ways by a vast variety of people with ideas and theories, some able to see the energy, some not, some sensing it, not all knowing what they are sensing or seeing. Not all of them have connected what they believe with their own inner sense of truth. They do not question, taking as truth what they hear or read, never studying the subject from their own experience to find their truth in what they sense and feel. Repeating ideas and theories as truths over decades does not make a truth. Many people who can see some of the aura doubt their own ability because it does not match what a so-called expert has said or written.

The aura is our record of our Earth life, our spirit energy and our link to our soul (see page 21). The aura record returns, with our spirit, to our soul when our physical body dies. The majority of people cannot see the aura in its entirety. They see parts of it sometimes, or cannot see it at all. They do not necessarily explain this, but communicate as though they are 'all-seeing'. Some who can see colours are unsure which layer of the aura they are seeing.

People register the aura energy in different ways. It is possible to sense the energy via the hands or to feel, in our own centres, the energy of another person. Most people 'sense' the aura rather than 'see' it.

All creatures use aura energy naturally to sense who is compatible and who is disturbing. This is a basic survival instinct and common to all. When we meet a person whom we feel ill-at-ease with, despite an attractive physical appearance, or others praising them, it is our aura energy which has made contact with theirs. It is letting us know we need to be on our guard or that it is safe to venture closer if the feeling is compatible. This effect can change on a later meeting if their, or our, energy changes. The incompatibility can be temporary; we may find we are still ill-at-ease at a second meeting. Tread with care in dealing with that person. It does not necessarily mean they are incompatible with others, or are necessarily a nasty person. If a feeling of well-being was present at first contact and remains at a later encounter, the person is compatible. Our first reaction is the one we should trust. We are all inclined to judge by appearance or pre-knowledge and allow this to interfere with the finer, unacknowledged aura sense.

If a person has a limb amputated, our physical eyes will not see a physical limb; however, their aura will still record the limb. The person will feel they have a physical limb long after it has been removed. Aura energy cannot be amputated. It has recorded a limb and will continue to do so for a very long time. Eventually the aura energy will fade in that part, but will never go away completely.

If a person is born without a limb, the aura will not be in evidence where that limb should be.

Aura energy can seem pale or intense, but it cannot disappear, be 'blocked' or have holes in it. It is complete and self-contained. All auras are different. While a person is alive, they have an aura field in and around their physical. When they die, it is no longer with their physical body; it belongs to and goes with the spirit. The silver/white second layer which is physical energy takes time to fade as the physical body winds down. This happens within hours.

THE SEVEN LAYERS

The aura consists of seven layers of pulsating, moving, many-coloured energy. It records on the various layers all we have done, dream of, hope for; our potential, health, weaknesses and strengths; whom we have known, know now, where we have lived, and what we have achieved. It constantly clears and cleans itself of unwanted energy, but the record remains intact. When we involuntarily shake or shiver, we are clearing unwanted matter from our aura, just as animals do when they leave the company of humans.

If we leave our body when asleep, a proportion of the aura will go with the spirit on its travels. The silver/white glow, which is the second layer, is electro-magnetic and is created by our physical body energy. This layer is always with the living body, whether the spirit is present or on its travels. The part of the centre colours which are the first layer and relate to our internal organ energy will also remain but will seem fainter. These colours are part of the spirit, but are vital to the well-being of the physical as well, and so continue to reflect our health and well-being while all other colours will remain with the spirit wherever it goes. If a spirit is away from the body and anything happens to, or approaches near the body, either by energy, noise or touch, the energies will immediately signal the spirit to return and protect its physical existence.

If we are physically low in energy, the second layer will appear dull. If we are high in energy, this layer will shine and glow. Our physical energy shown in the second silver/white layer is very like a battery. It increases with use, but becomes sluggish and dull through lack of action, mentally or physically. A person who is continuously resting is not conserving energy, they are no longer creating it. The longer we remain still, mentally or physically, the harder it becomes to move or think when we are ready to do so.

On occasions, the aura needs an energy boost. This depletion can be caused through illness, stress, incompatible company and/or environment. A healer is able to supply the energy needed, giving the person what they need to begin creating their own energy in order to heal themselves.

The complete aura is equally high, wide and deep around our physical body. It is seen as an oval or flame-shape with the body in the centre. If two people are standing close to each other, they will sense difference of energies. When they part, they will naturally clear any exchange which has occurred. If we remain near or in the company of people who are depressed, angry, frightened, or intense, we can, after a while, attract their energy pattern from their physical electric layer to ourselves. It will be drawn into our electro-magnetic energy and can affect our well-being and personality. Leaving the

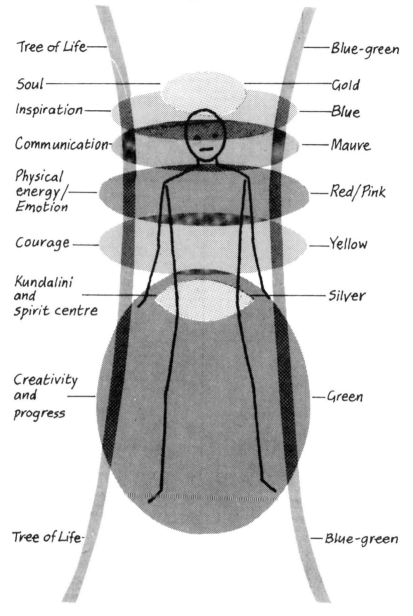

Tree of Life —————— Blue-green
Soul —————————————— Gold
Inspiration ————— Blue
Communication— ————— Mauve
Physical energy/ —— Red/Pink
Emotion
Courage ————— Yellow
Kundalini and spirit centre ————— Silver
Creativity and progress ——— Green
Tree of Life— —Blue-green

The Different Centres and Colours in the Aura

presence of the other person and clearing the aura will remove the effect, returning to them will increase it. This is physical energy level attraction.

The first layer of the aura is the innermost one and very colourful. It is often thought to be the second layer, which it shines through, and appears to be outside.

The first layer has the same colours, plus overlap colours, for all of us. Each colour is based and remains in its own centre, but is also represented in all other centres as it pulses through them and back to its own space. Each centre colour changes in shade according to the well-being (physical and spiritual) of a person.

These centres respond to the energies of various sounds, stones, quartz, metal, shapes, number energy, emotions, environment, planets and people.

FIRST LAYER

Working from the head downwards, the energy centres are as follows:

Soul connection centre

Gold

This centre is the soul connection and is based in the top of the head. The gold can expand until it shines above and around the head when we are in harmony or in contact with our soul. The soul centre is never overlapped by other centres. It is within the blue centre but is apart from it.

Colour:	Gold	Number energy: 1
Star:	Sun	

Metal: Gold
Shape: ‿

Inspiration – Head centre

Blue

This centre is based in the upper half of the head and seen around it. The colour is a deep shade of blue when we are content and mentally balanced. It can deepen in colour and widen in size when we are inspired. When we are depressed this centre is immediately affected. The colour can intensify until it looks black and can be seen as a dark cloud around head and shoulders.

Some depressions weaken the blue and, as it moves through other centres via its connecting line, it can give the impression that the person is blue. We have common sayings about this, i.e. 'I have my own personal black cloud' or 'I feel blue.'

Colour: Blue   Number energy: 8
Planet: Saturn
Quartz: Sapphire
Shape: ✡

Communication – Throat centre

Mauve

This centre is concentrated around the lower head including ears, mouth and the neck. The mauve is deep, but not intense when we are able to communicate with others and ourselves. Should we be in contact with our spirit and soul, the colour deepens to purple. It also deepens in shade if we are speaking with emotion or conviction. If we are unable to communicate, the colour can become heavy and the throat constrict, or it can become very pale giving us an all-over glow of coolness which does not attract others to communicate. In our speech we have the saying: 'Purple prose'.

Colour: Mauve   Number energy: 7
Planet: Mercury
Quartz: Amethyst
Shape: ≈≈

Emotional and physical – Heart centre

Pink/Red
These colours surround the heart centre and can be seen from the top of shoulders, down to the middle of the ribs including the arms and hands. The energy is affected by physical and emotional patterns.

Pink
This is the colour of emotion. It is a deep pink when in harmony and when we are cared for, loved or loving, and shines around us as a pink glow. When we feel unloved or unable to love, the pink becomes paler and we appear dull and do not attract others in the way we would like to. The arms can lose strength if caring contact is not made.

Red
This is the colour of physical energy. A person who is strong in action and determination will have a rosy glow. This physical energy is also connected to hatred and resentment. The red energy can rise as anger when we lose our temper. In our common language we say: 'I see red' when we are angry. The physical can become

bright red around the neck and ears as the energy rises. The emotions of love and hate are the extremes in this double centre and one can overshadow the other, or turn from one to the other very easily as the centre energies combine and interrelate.

	Emotion	*Physical*
Colours:	Pink	Red
Planets:	Pluto	Mars
Quartz:	Rose	Ruby
Shape:	✕	▢
And combine into:	⊠	
Number energy:	5	4

Courage and security – Solars centre

Yellow

The courage centre is based in what is also called the solar area, which is from half-way down the ribs to the top of the hips. It is seen as a deep yellow inner ring and a lighter yellow outer ring. It is the security and courage centre. When we are strong and secure in our life patterns, this centre glows like the sun and we feel tall and unafraid.

However, if we are insecure or afraid, the yellow changes. Insecurity causes the colour to become dull and weak. Fear or terror can intensify the colour and we look yellow as it permeates all our centres. It affects our stomach, kidneys, liver, bladder and bowels. This centre is constantly sensing other people and all energies from outside, and reflects our inner and outer strength of purpose. In our common language we say a coward is 'yellow' or call them 'a yellow belly'.

Colour: Yellow   Number energy: 2
Planet: Jupiter
Resin: Amber/
            inner ring
Quartz: Yellow Topaz/
            outer ring
Shape: ⊚

Creativity and progress – Creative centre

Green

This centre is based in the lower body from the top of the hips down to the bottom of the feet. It is a deep green and when we are creative in any way, progressing in our own time through life, it is in harmony. If, however, we are envious or jealous, the green can intensify and pain can be felt in this area. If we feel unable to progress for any reason, our legs can become weak. In our common language we say: 'Green with envy' or 'Green with jealousy'. When we indulge in these emotions we become a sickly green.

Colour: Green   Number energy: 3
Planet: Venus
Quartz: Emerald
Shape: ▽

Tree of Life – Nerve centre

Deep green/blue

This centre is based at the core of our physical body beginning above our head and finishing beneath our feet. From this centre, fine, fern-like energy, tipped with silver, reaches out and permeates all other centres. It is affected by our physical and emotional well-being. If we are nervous for any reason, or have a nerve-affecting illness, the connection of this centre energy is weakened. Each centre is based on this tree of life energy and they all feed and affect each other via the tree. This energy will cause us to quiver and shake, to become immovable, or run in panic when we become nervous. It can become so weak we have a total nervous breakdown, as it is unable to energise all the other centres.

Colour: Green/blue   Number energy: 10
Planets: Uranus/Neptune
Stones: Jade/turquoise
Shape:)(

Spirit centre

Silvery/white
This centre is also called Kundalini. It is the energy base our spirit links in to for replenishment and connection to all our other centres. It is located at the base of our spine and, similar to the soul centre, it is self-contained inasmuch as it does not overlap other centres, even though it is near to the creative centre. This is a centre like all others. Often it is written and said that this centre should not be activated, tuned into or otherwise used, unless someone who professes to know takes us through careful initiations and knowledge which we are told can take years. However, it is impossible not to have active centres. They all connect and affect each other whether we do anything purposeful about them or not. To deny this centre its rightful place on our tree of life is like asking a strong healthy plant to grow and expand without its roots,

or to expect a machine to work with its electricity supply turned off or down. We need to activate and expand our energies. To ignore an energy centre undernourishes it.

All our centres are functionable at all times. Fear is the greatest enemy we have; it can be passed to us by others and/or we can create and feed it. We can remove fear by debate and questions, reaching an understanding of ourselves. When we remove our fears we become aware and tune into our strengths. As mentioned before, our spirit is our life-force while on Earth. Our soul is our true self, always in contact with our spirit via our soul centre. We do not all give attention to our spiritual needs or acknowledge our inner self. When we seek knowledge, we can find a way through our fear. Be very careful to check all information given, to avoid being filled with old, worn, unproven ideas which repress and suppress human greatness; investigate and cross-check, do not be put off by frighteners who say acknowledging this centre is dangerous, or only for the few, to be awakened by a certain person, and so on.

Colour: Silvery/white   Number energy: 9
Planet: Moon
Stone: Moonstone
Shape: ⬭

Halo

Multicoloured
Around the head is a band of light consisting of all the centre colours and similar to a rainbow effect. It does not relate to specifics as it is the reflection of all the centre colours in the brain, which controls the

organs and workings of the physical body. When we are in tune with life, at peace with our spirit and soul, we are in harmony and this band glows. It is sometimes called a halo. Because it is really a reflection of all centre energies in the brain, it is not a true centre.

Overlap colours

The overlap colours are between the centres:

- blue and mauve;
- mauve, pink and red;
- pink, red and yellow;
- yellow and green.

1 When we are inspired and able to communicate inwardly and outwardly, the blue and mauve overlap deepens. If we are depressed, the overlap becomes darker or pale, communication becomes difficult and the overlap colour can become so deep it appears almost black.

2 When we are energetic and emotionally strong, the mauve, pink and red overlap becomes bright and vibrant. We communicate through this energy, by word or deed. If we are emotionally unhappy, we talk too much or become silent and withdrawn. When anger is present, the red combines strongly with the mauve, causing head and heart palpitations and we look darkly bruised. We shout and storm or brood and become menacing.

3 When we are secure and unafraid, the overlap of yellow with the red and pink appears as a deep golden-pink. Should we be disturbed emotionally

and fearful, this band appears orange. Hyperactive people can be violent due to the overlap of fear, emotional instability and resentment. All things orange should be removed from them to enable the aura to achieve balance.

4 When we are creative and progressing steadily, the overlap of green and yellow is bright and strong. It looks like the colour of new grass. When we are jealous, envious or fearful about life and progress, the overlap becomes a muddy yellowy-green.

Performers, which include politicians, orators, preachers, actors, singers, etc., can activate the energy of all their centres when they work. They can feel inspired, creative, emotional, strong and communicative. This causes them to become attractive and magnetic; they shine. They can attract a following of people quite out of proportion to the quality, content or truth of what they are involved in or believe.

SECOND LAYER

The second layer of the aura is the physical electromagnetic energy. It appears as a white glow next to the skin around the entire body. The first layer already mentioned shines through and can reflect its colours on this layer.

All living things have this brightness around them, whether it be water, mountains, humans, creatures of land, sea and air, plants, stones or quartz. All life-forms vibrate and create electro magnetic energy.

In relation to humans, the second layer is an indication of our physical energy balances. When we are listening

intently, speaking, gesticulating, moving head, shoulders
or arms, the energy will intensify around the upper body.
If we are running, walking or otherwise physically using
our lower body, the energy will glow brightly in that area.
When we are still it will seem less bright.

This layer is magnetic. It draws from the aura all
energies which are unnatural to it. For example: if a
person who is well-balanced spends a lot of time with, or
watches and listens to, people who are unhappy, disturbed,
fearful or working against the well-being of others, they
can gradually attract and receive these vibrations. The
energy pattern will be drawn through their aura to this
second layer where it will settle and affect their harmony
and personality. Shaking the body will remove most of
this unwanted energy, and clearing of the aura will
remove the rest.

A complete personality change can take place when
these energy patterns are allowed to remain. It is natural
for this second layer to clear itself of unwanted energy patterns and it does this by causing us to shiver or shake.

Whenever a person shivers or shakes for no apparent
reason, it is highly likely their aura is shaking off
unwanted vibrations. If another person is sending strong
anti-energies and thought-forms, it is this layer of aura
which will attract them, but will shake them off, as long
as the recipient allows this process. We can become
afraid when we feel out of tune or believe that others
can harm us by energy thought-patterns, believing we
have no choice in the matter. We therefore hang on
to the energy received instead of releasing it through a
good shake and refusing to be affected. Physical action
removes unwanted energies.

No-one can be affected by another person sending
energy or thought-forms, if they refuse that energy.

Only our fear and ignorance allow it to stick like glue and affect us. A brisk walk, a shower, a swim, any physically strong movement will clear the mind and aura and will help remove or repel energy attracted or sent, which is unwanted.

OTHER LAYERS

The other layers of aura energy record all we have done, are doing, or have the capacity to do. They also record all the people we have known and places we have been, everything that has happened to and around us.

The aura is a record coded as colour. It does not have pictures in it, but a psychic can pick up vibrations from the aura layers of another person, and sense or see them as words or pictures. The way the psychic translates the information is of the utmost importance, as what they see or sense can be read in many ways, and needs careful presentation. The information received is to help people heal themselves and progress in their own way. The information is often symbolic as well as factual.

These layers are always different on each person. We cannot have the same record, however close we may be in life. All colours are represented through the aura and can be translated according to where they are sensed or seen.

For example:

Orange: as an overlap in the first layer, it is a sign of fear and emotional disturbance. Orange seen in other layers can mean liveliness and integration.

Blue: in various shades, other than the inspiration centre, also relates to honesty and outer harmony. Blue is also used to heal bones.

Green: relates to inner harmony and intunement and a love of life and nature, as well as creativity and progress.

Pink: is used to heal flesh wounds and also shows a carer of animals, as well as being the colour of emotion.

The appreciation of the depth and variety of colours in the aura obviously depends on the ability of the psychic viewing them. Psychics sense on different levels, and some are not able to 'see' colour at all.

It is not easy to describe aura colours to others who cannot see them as the whole structure is mobile and changeable at all times. Although the innermost layer and the second electro-magnetic layer retain the same colour, they also can fluctuate in depth of shade and reach. The colours are not solid, they are translucent.

Every aura is different because people are different. We respond to energy patterns around us wherever or whatever causes them, but we do not have to hold on to them.

All colours are represented in the aura, no colour being better or worse than another. It is the depth of colour which indicates the balance of a person. Colour is energy, energy is neither good nor bad. Humans affect energy and cause imbalances.

Some colours in the aura can seem to be unacceptable if read according to our preconceived ideas. For instance, black is often interpreted as something bad or evil, when in reality black is an energy and has meanings. It is, for example, the colour of the inner self, the deep unknown.

From childhood we have been taught that black is bad and white is good. This has become part of our subconscious and affects our view of people. When an inner aura colour is darkened by intensity to seem black, help is needed. If black is sensed in the outer aura, it means the person is reaching into and out from their inner self to gain clarity and knowledge. White is the outer self, the seeable.

When a person, adult or child, has had a shock or feels insecure, they will often wear black or paint or draw in black. This is a sign they are reaching inside themselves to their spirit for comfort and warmth, which they cannot find outside themselves. They wear the colour or paint with it to symbolise this.

When the outer, seeable, world is not felt to be giving comfort or understanding, we reach naturally inside to the darkness and comfort of our inner being, trying to find answers in order to see our way clearly in the outer life. This is why many people wear black, or draw in black, because they are lost and are seeking security. When they feel secure and braver they will gradually bring colour into their outer life and drawings.

If a person is forced to wear colours, or paint and draw in colours, before they are naturally able to do so, they will become more withdrawn. By showing their darkness, they release their despair and find help, eventually being able to move on in life at their own pace.

Grey is a colour we associate with dullness, sadness and grief. When seen in the aura, it can be a sign of a need for calm and peace. If it is seen around the shoulders and tinged with pink, it is a sign of being loved or loving in a calm and comforting way.

A reddish-brown seen around the lower body area shows the person is in touch with life and is well based. When seen around the head, it shows they are out of touch with physical life and are seeking inspiration.

When a healer is working with a person, their own aura can become more deeply coloured and bright because of the energy that is moving through them to the person in need. It is not the energy of the other person, but the healing energy going via the healer to that person.

Part IV

Ceremonies

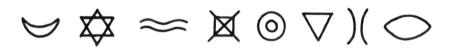

Ceremonies

Through the ages, humankind has devised many rituals and ceremonies to make certain occasions outstanding and memorable. Some of these celebrations were statements and brought harmony, joy and understanding to all. Combining energies in the presence of friends and those we care for gives an added dimension to our existence as physical beings and links the energies of the spirit and soul to our earthly life. The following ceremonies incorporate the four elements as then known and considered vital for health and happiness: Air, Fire, Water and Earth. We can use these ceremonies, with slight adaptions, in our lives now.

28
The Joining Ceremony

The Joining Ceremony is used when two people have decided to acknowledge their decision to live as a partnership, and want all those they care for to know and join in the celebration. This ceremony enables energies from all those present to contribute to the occasion and gives each person an opportunity to link with their own dreams and aspirations. The energy combination on these occasions is very moving emotionally and spiritually and delights the soul.

Needed:
1 *an arch made* of wood, about 8 ft high (?½ m) at its centre, covered with flowers, branches and herbs, placed on the earth, near water in the open air; this is where the couple sit;
2 *six fire-sticks, candles or lights* placed on the earth, spaced equally in front of the arch in a circle;
3 *flowers* placed between the fire-sticks on the earth in arcs, bowing outwards;
4 *baskets of flower petals and herbs;*

5 *chairs* for two people under the arch; for three
speakers and one co-ordinator, each side of the
arch; and for guests, facing the arch, within the
circle, leaving a space between these chairs and
the arch;
6 *music or musicians* behind the arch;
7 a place for the feasting and dancing after the
ceremony.

Each partner chooses in advance three people to speak
for them. At the ceremony these friends talk about the
couple and recommend them to each other, or play
music, recite, sing, anything which is joyful. They take
turns, one from each side. A co-ordinator is selected to
conduct the ceremony, indicating by a nod of the head
whose turn it is to speak, after they have spoken themselves and explained what the ceremony represents and
how all present are part of it.

When all is ready, the fire-sticks are lit, the music
begins and the guests form two rows, from the circle
to the water (which can be natural or bowls of water)
from where the couple are going to begin their walk and,
as they reach the corridor of guests, children scatter the
petals and herbs, from the baskets, in front of them.
The couple walk between the rows of guests who then
in twos, walk behind the couple, so that a procession
forms back to the arch. The children sit in front of the
guests. The couple sit under the arch, the six speakers
and co-ordinator sit each side and the guests sit in rows
facing the couple (see page 172).

The co-ordinator opens the proceedings and the six
friends take turns to speak or perform. The couple tell
the company how they met and grew to the stage of
wanting to be together. They then talk to each other, of

171

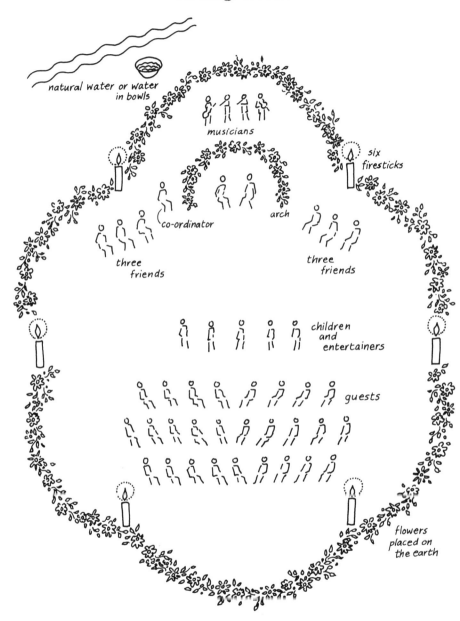

natural water or water
in bowls

musicians

six
firesticks

arch

co-ordinator

three
friends

three
friends

children
and
entertainers

guests

flowers
placed on
the earth

Plan for Ceremonies

their love and care, relating their dreams and hopes for their future together. They exchange rings or gifts. The children and performers then entertain the company in the space between the couple and the guests.

When all is complete the couple walk from the arch out of the circle, followed by the children, the co-ordinator, four of the friends, and all the guests to the celebration venue.

The remaining friends (with willing helpers) put out the fire-sticks and, if the celebration is to be held indoors, clear the site. They then join the others.

29
The Naming Ceremony

Bestowing the energy of a name for use during this life on a child is a necessary and important occasion. The name should be chosen for its energy flow when it is spoken out loud, i.e. a rhythm in the full name including the surname inherited from its parents.

When a child is ready to receive its names for its stay on Earth, a ceremony is used called the Naming Ceremony. The same setting is used as for the Joining Ceremony, including the six friends and co-ordinator. When the fire-sticks are lit, the parent(s) walk to the arch, from the water, carrying the child, through the columns of guests who follow them to their seats.

The co-ordinator explains the ceremony. The six friends speak in turn about the parent(s) and the world the child will live in, and welcome it to the planet or, if they prefer they can recite or make music. The parent(s) then speak to the child and tell of their hopes and dreams for the future. They thank the child for choosing them, saying how they intend to care, love, cherish, and be its guardians.

They then hold the child between them and, lifting it as high as they can towards the moon or sun, they say clearly:

> As he/she was
> As he/she is
> As he/she will be
> I (we) name this child...

They will then sit with the child, under the arch, and the children or entertainers perform. Finally the parent(s) and child leave the circle and, followed by the guests, go to the place of celebration and feasting. The friends clear the site and join them.

These two ceremonies are not the property of any one group, but of all people. They overcome boundaries of different beliefs, cultures, backgrounds and needs. They create beauty and harmony among people.

30
The Parting Ceremony

When the energies exchanged in a partnership become destructive instead of constructive, and when the together times are no longer a pleasure and joy but are dreaded, or the energies between the partners fade to a level which is pleasant but not sustaining enough, it is time to reassess. If necessary a Parting ceremony is convened in order to state that the partners are no longer choosing to combine their energies and to enable friends and family to come to terms with the fact that the couple have chosen to become single again. This can also be carried out if only one of the partners wants to attend.

The arch, fire, earth and air setting are used, as already explained. The couple walk through the column of friends and stand under the arch, their friends and family seated before them. There are no speakers, but six friends who can recite or make music can be present to support them. The co-ordinator explains what is happening.

The couple thank each other for the good times, apologise where it is needed and ask friends and family to understand and be kind to them as singles. They give each other a farewell gift or return their rings. If only one of the partnership is present they tell the guests why it is wise that they are no longer with their partner.

When this is completed, they walk from the circle, one to the left, one to the right. They are now welcomed into the company of their friends and family as singles, and a celebration of food and music begins.

This ceremony removes the embarrassment of not knowing of the parting, and enables all to understand. Friendships cannot be cut in half because two people part; they have to accommodate the new status of the two people concerned.

31
The
Festival of
Light Ceremony

Another ceremony from the past is the Festival of Light. It originated because in the winter the sun appeared to be leaving the planet and the energies of the land were less active and sustaining. The people feared the sun would not return and re-energise the Earth and, in so doing, re-energise them. They made fires on hilltops and in valleys which they kept alight for eight days to entice the sun to return and stay.

After the eighth day it appears as though the sun has seen the light of the fires and decides to return. It was seen as the rebirth of life. In the British Isles, this time occurs from 21 December to 28 December inclusive.

This ceremony has been adopted knowingly or unknowingly by many beliefs and religions. During the Festival of Light we honour the past because we are the past; the present because we are the present; and the future because we are the future. We cannot blame those who went before or ignore those who will follow. We are the now. Life is ours. We are here and share every breath we breathe, every word we say and every thought energy we release. Each of us is a contributor. If we do not honour the ongoing life of the planet, we have no base to see how far we have progressed, as individuals and collectively, or to see where we are, or how much our influence will affect the future.

When 21 December arrives the Festival of Light begins and we light a candle every day for eight days; two days to honour our past, four days to assess our present and two days to contemplate our hopes for the future, of ourselves as individuals and the world as a whole.

32
The
Seasons

In time gone by when people lived in small communities they acknowledged the strength of their combined energy, their surroundings and honoured them. They performed plays to fit the seasons of nature and the passing of time. This helped them to understand and cope with change in their own life patterns; birth, youth, middle years, old age and death.

Certain people were designated guardians of the knowledge and ceremony and made sure all people in the communities joined together on special days for the life plays, the work required and the fun afterwards, honouring a particular nature essence and folklore story in doing so. These customs are now being revived and the work expanded to include modern life. Some people are reawakening the memories of the plays for the seasons while others honour the need to care for the environment.

| Spring | Spirit of Water |
| Summer | Spirit of Air |

The Seasons

| Autumn | Spirit of Earth |
| Winter | Spirit of Fire |

On a designated day in spring, the Spirit of Water was honoured. Everyone, the very young to the very old, joined together to clear up all streams, canals, rivers and waterways of debris and silt build-up. Nowadays we could include checking and clearing all water tanks and water supply systems, and include checking waste water from domestic and industrial premises. All water and its containers of whatever use could be checked for cleanliness. We would also check ourselves to see our own water energies run clearly and freely.

In summer, a day was dedicated to the Spirit of Air. Today we could check that all sprays are safe for the ozone layer, all smells are sweet, gases and smoke from all chimneys checked for pollution, personally seeing that our homes are clean and smell pleasant, and that our body odours and breath are not offensive. Radiation levels should be checked. We could also check our breathing patterns, our lungs and clear our own airways.

In autumn a day was spent in honour of the Spirit of Earth. All people would do something collectively or separately to turn the soil and clear the Earth of objects which were unsightly or causing a blockage. Today we could collect all waste from the streets, parks or homes. Those who need to could use the time to clear their minds of clutter and fear. Digging, drain unblocking, gardening, all could be tackled on this day. We could also look at our physical health as a whole.

Which brings us to the Spirit of Fire which was honoured in winter by collecting and storing wood for fires to cook by and keep warm, mending homes and fences, checking places where fire was used. Today we could

181

clean chimneys of soot and deposits, check electric and gas fires, cookers, central heating systems, all electrical appliances, fire-fighting equipment and so on. We could also check our physical energy, or lack of it.

Obviously all the work needed cannot be completed in one day, but the fact that all people join together in a common cause for one day forges friendships and reveals unused abilities. It also makes people more aware and more committed to a clean environment, recognising the value of people who do the work all year round. It also makes us aware of our own bodies and the condition we are in.

If we start in a small way, taking one bank holiday in a season to do all we can for the essence of that season, everyone from the young to the old can join in combining energy instead of sitting alone, or creating discord.

Part V

Questions and Answers

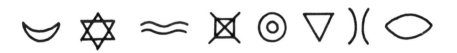

Questions and Answers

Questions are life, their energy comes from the questioner who can be speaking unknowingly on behalf of many others – in effect a community energy can be behind any question. Some questions recur and are often debated and written about. The following are some of these.

Does consciousness and memory continue after physical death?

Consciousness belongs to the spirit and therefore stays with the spirit at physical death, but the memories of the life just left become less and less as the spirit becomes integrated with its soul. The experiences of the physical life then become part of the soul memory, which includes memories of experiences from all past physical lives.

Can soul integration be held up by memories of physical life attachments and does the memory of people loved and left behind interfere with the absorption of the spirit?

If a person has physical attachments, either to material possessions or people, when they leave the physical life as a spirit, they retain the memory of that attachment. As the spirit is absorbed by its soul, so the memories mellow and take on new meanings. The memories do not interfere with soul integration, but ~~unitl~~ all the last *until* physical life attachments are clarified and understood, the spirit cannot be absorbed. We meet and communicate on many levels on earth, but when the spirit returns to its soul, it returns to reality and re-unites with the true life energy and memory. Any attachments from the physical life gradually ease into the soul life. The needs and emotions of the physical body fade as the soul absorbs the memories the spirit has returned with. Love is no longer obsessive or possessive. The memory of the Earth attachment would mellow and all memories become part of the complete experience.

Does our soul choose our partners on Earth before we begin our new life experience?

This pre-arrangement is very rare. It is not usual to choose partners in advance. We need a partner who is an extension and/or an opposite of ourselves while we are physical spiritual beings. All people grow and change and also spiritually expand during a lifetime. Each spirit energy comes from a different soul and souls exist on many levels of refinement. Physical people are attracted to each other for various reasons including sexual, emotional, visual and spiritual. We change our energy when we spend time with a person in a partnership. Choosing a partner before birth would pre-suppose that physically and spiritually we will reach a specific energy point at the same time, whatever happens in our life, which would mean we were totally programmed in advance. This rules out choice, which is essential for growth on all levels.

The spirit knows what is needed while on Earth and strives to place itself, in its physical body, in a position where it can experience, physically and spiritually, learning on all levels, to be of benefit to itself, others and the planet. At times we attract certain people and become attracted to them. This is an Earth choice and they become part of our experience.

Do parents choose the soul energy of their children, or does the soul choose the parents? Why are the choices made?

The choice is made by the soul. When it is ready to experience physical Earth life via its spirit energy, it becomes aware of what is possible from certain physical connections, and the type of life its spirit energy would most likely experience in the first seven years. Souls would know the situation of the people they choose and their likely projection. Once the child is able to reason, the spirit will constantly try to see the best way for itself to expand. We are not programmed in advance for life. If we remove choice from our existence, we remove growth. The day we are born begins our experience of this life. The soul receives information from its spirit energy but cannot directly interfere. The physical inheritance of the parents is part of the physical life of the new child, and the spirit energy within the child will try to absorb this inheritance in order to expand and make choices.

Does a soul choose and a woman conceive or does a woman conceive and the soul choose? Some people are born into a very stressful and hard life. Surely the soul does not choose this?

The soul has the choice of where it will place its spirit energy for a life on Earth. A soul which has chosen to experience a physical existence via its spirit energy connects with the life energy as conception occurs. Souls tune into the area they have chosen to be born into, or the parents most suitable for the physical background of their spirit energy. Because all conceptions need spirit energy in order to have life, and the pattern of life is strong, some souls connect even in the direst circumstances, knowing the situation will be very difficult. Those choices of a life on Earth incorporate the need to bring to the attention of all of us on Earth the lack of care or support others have, and encourages those better situated to care and practise guardianship of all in need. On Earth we share the physical experience. If we help each other we raise the quality of life for all. We have the ability, via our spirit energy, to remove our fears and achieve a sense of Oneness without losing our individuality.

Do multiple births, twins, for instance, share a spirit?

No. Each of us has a different spirit energy from a different soul. Twins can share an egg which is physical, but not a soul or spirit energy. Each spirit has its own path to follow and each soul seeks completeness. While on Earth we individually seek awareness on all three levels of life, physical, spiritual and soul.

What do we leave on Earth when our physical body dies?

While we live on Earth we leave memories of ourselves wherever we go and with whomever we meet. All action creates energy and when we help others, as individuals or as groups, we help others to help themselves. If we work to improve living conditions for others, we should ask what is needed, show technique if required and give the help required. This creates the energy and interest in others to do more. The memory of the persons who instigated the help will remain. The fact that people have offered help and care stays in the memory of those concerned long afterwards. Memory is impressed in the aura record, in the atmosphere and in buildings. Meeting in certain places to combine energy, to send to those in need, creates a memory. We can feel energy in a room or place. It does not fade if it is energised by others, and lasts forever if people care enough to add to it.

The energy of memory is being created by each of us, all the time. Memories enable people and events to live on in the minds of humankind. When a person physically dies and people want to remember them, they try to recall details, searching their memories for things that happened. If a parent dies, the children will say to each other: 'Do you remember when they took us to . . .?' and an old, cherished memory is recalled. People live on in memories and if we bring those memories forward they are energised and live on. They fade, but do not disappear. Even when people no longer recall them, they are printed on the combined consciousness of humankind for all time.

When we attend meetings, groups, or are involved in an event, we each attend for a different reason. Each person is affected in a different way and by their recall of the event. If we are involved in something wonderful, even for a moment, we cannot be the same again; that good moment has now become a part of our memory and energy and we have an added quality.

It is better to recall the memory of one bright moment, than a dozen feeble ones. A good memory shared is a beautiful gift. Meeting a person who recalls a wonderful experience can affect us; the whole day can light up and there is a sparkle around. We may see or hear something by chance which warms us, a face, a scene which keeps recurring perhaps for days, that makes such a glowing impression the memory lives on. If we visit a place and feel in harmony, we leave good vibrations and memories far outlasting our trip.

Obviously we also leave and retain unhappy or frightening memories. There can be situations where people have promised help, begin to visit and do not return. The person in need remembers the promise and a sad memory is registered. When someone cares, the energy is light, the memory is strong.

Unfortunately, sad and traumatic memories are registered as strongly as good ones, and also affect us all. As we all leave behind memories of ourselves while we live and when we leave, we should be a little more careful what those memories are!

Do we bring particular past life imbalances with us to clear or overcome in the current life, meeting people we knew before whom we badly treated, or were badly treated by, to redress the past?

Humankind at different levels has been in existence on Earth for millions of years and our soul, our true self, has been steadily progressing through all that time. The progress and refinement of the soul includes experiencing a multitude of lives on Earth. It is what we do in this life and how we conduct ourselves which is important; we cannot relive the past.

Life is an ongoing experience of the soul, which is immortal. Our lives on Earth as physical beings are part of that evolution of the soul and each life is dealt with, assessed and absorbed by the soul, before a return to a life on Earth is possible. Each life is complete, irrespective of what happened or how long or short it was.

We are born into a new life on Earth to write another chapter. We cannot rewrite what is already recorded. The soul will tune into its spirit on Earth with ideas, compassion, encouragement, clues and memories of experiences that have been recorded from past lives, but not as a punishment. We do not return to Earth to clear up past lives or repeat them, but we do trigger memories from our soul of experience gained when necessary.

To our soul each past life is like a day to us in this life. Our present life will seem like a day when we return to our soul at the end of this life. The art of life is to live each day fully, using the past for experience, planning for the future. We can use past lives for experience, but cannot repeat them. We cannot be five years old again in this life, any more than we can be a person we were in a past life.

A past life is experience gained to be used, not lived again. We cannot repeat anything exactly as it was. All persons and situations have moved on and changed. When we link into a memory or pattern of a past life which has been triggered by our circumstances now, instead of using the knowledge to overcome the reason, some use it as an excuse for feelings and reactions to others they meet.

Some people believe they stay as the last person they were on Earth and that that person is walking around somewhere in the heavens until it is time to return to Earth, then the same person is born here again. This is not so. Think of continuance: nothing remains the same. As souls, we are an accumulation of knowledge, events and experiences.

A life is a fragment of that whole soul self. When the spirit energy comes to Earth for a physical life experience, it is to meet other spirit energies representing souls from all levels of evolution. Earth is the only place that spirit energy from various levels of soul, however different they are, can meet together and communicate and this is because we share the same physical body vibration through which to function. As souls we live at the level of energy we have achieved. It is very difficult for the soul to function on the level of another vibration. The soul sees living on Earth as a vital experience where sharing, caring and learning is for all. We are here to help each other and the planet. We all breathe the same air and are part of a vast energy pattern. Each of us is highly individual, but seeking not to become individualistic.

Many people have resigned themselves to misery, having been told their experiences and hardships are a result of their behaviour in a past life. Instead of checking the cause of their trouble in their present life and dealing with it, they accept it as a punishment. Using past lives as excuses removes the choice of our actions now. We create our own destiny as we live and choose day by day.

In finding out why we are behaving in a certain way, we may pick up on a past-life memory, not because we are re-living or being punished by a past life. We cannot deal with past lives in the present because we are not the physical person or at the same spiritual level we were in another life. Our environment is different, as are our parents and genetic inheritance; our education; the food we eat; everything about us is totally different. The soul progresses at all times whether an Earth life is involved or not.

What is acceptable or not acceptable in one life on Earth could be totally reversed in a later incarnation. Different ages and social structures dictate different ways of living and acceptance. Taking historical facts out of context and trying to judge them as we now are is an imbalance, and so is taking a past life out of context and judging it in the present.

The soul does not release a spirit energy of itself into a life on Earth until it has cleared the last life. We come to Earth to experience, through learning and teaching, to help each other, to refine, and to care for the planet.

One of our reasons for being on Earth is to raise the combined consciousness of humankind by improving our behaviour to each other, and all life, to a higher level of humanity.

Our personal day-by-day problems are important while we are on Earth, but not so important when our body has died and the spirit is back with its soul, striving to become integrated. The issues affecting the life we have been involved in are very important, as we all affect the lives of others. All have to be assessed and attempts made to gain understanding and clarity.

As with our past lives, so with our present life; understanding and forgiving of ourselves is important. We should not continually beat ourselves for things we did when we were younger, in a different environment, with different teachers, different circumstances.

We have to acknowledge we behaved that way because of those circumstances and lack of understanding. Try and correct if possible, but if not absorb and move on. All we do is part of us and nothing can be removed from our life record, or from our soul record.

Sometimes we can find ourselves in situations which create a space for us to behave in an unacceptable way. When we are young, we are very vulnerable and lacking wisdom. We are bombarded from all directions with sights, sounds, ideas. On occasions we join groups because they are different, or experiment and get addicted in mind or body. Some fight for ideals which are not their own because they are too young and inexperienced to understand. These times in our life are part of growing and understanding. All we have been through as we go through life is part of our whole person, and therefore valid, as it makes us what we are. We can always assess and adjust if we really want to. So it is with past lives.

It is not possible for us to forgive or be forgiven without understanding. We have to be able to forgive ourselves. That is the hardest of all. Someone else giving forgiveness does not have a meaning unless we can forgive ourselves. When we have wronged someone, we need to get understanding from them and not repeat our action. Understanding is all we can ask for and that can be hard to get. A person can say they forgive without fully understanding our action. If they try, or do understand why we behaved as we did, progress is possible on both sides.

When our spirit returns to its soul at death, it is given the opportunity to meet with the spirits of those about whom it feels incomplete and who are still alive. While they are physically asleep, their spirit energies can meet and try to gain understanding of why, in the physical life, certain actions occurred.

The living person very often wakes up, having had a dream about meeting the person who has died, remembering the conversation and explanation and finding hatred and fear have receded and a peace is in its place. We often hear people say they went to sleep hating someone and, in the morning, felt it was pointless to feel that way as it did not matter any more. We live in the now and do not live in past lives.

The spirit cannot be absorbed into its soul until there is harmony between them. The disharmonies of the last life have to be cleared. Some spirits have to wait until the person they need understanding from has died and their spirit returned to its soul before understanding is achieved. The spirit may be willing while on Earth, but the brain memory unable to accept and release the painful experiences. We cannot return to this planet until all past experiences have been accepted and cleared. We do not come back as the same person, but as an energy of our soul. Our soul never comes to Earth. The spirit we are today is a part of the whole soul and can tune into the experiences and memories of past existence. To believe that we bring back to Earth a list of particular past-life actions means the record we bring back will not relate to the spirit energy we are, because it is from another experience, another self, another time, another place, and has all been completed before our return as another energy.

We change continually as physical beings and spiritual soul beings. Some souls choose to have a physical experience, via the spirit energy, in the same location. This is not to repeat a life, but because the pull of energy to certain places is strong and attractive. On occasions, a short life on Earth can become a memory the soul wishes to explore further and a new life will begin very soon after the death of the last life. A spirit returning to its soul after a short life on Earth integrates very quickly.

Some souls send their spirit energy to Earth after ages have passed on Earth, some choose to return a few months later. It is totally up to the soul when its spirit energy returns. It will incorporate its own evolvement, the evolvement of the planet and the evolvement of other people. These are our three main purposes for a new life. If we look back at our present life we can see where one purpose has been more dominant than another.

If we share our experiences and knowledge, we can help someone else. If that knowledge prevents pollution of any kind of people on Earth, we are helping the planet. They all intermingle and intertwine. If we actually look at our life, we can see the threads weaving through each day and see what we are doing for each purpose. In each main purpose there are many personal purposes. Life is fascinating when we observe it and see how it all weaves together. We can then see where our choices are in this life, allowing the past to become experience gained just as we allow our past lives to become experience gained. It is a great loss to our present and future if we live in our past in this life, or through past lives.